MENTAL ILLNESS AND SOCIAL POLICY

The American Experience

MENTAL ILLNESS AND SOCIAL POLICY

THE AMERICAN EXPERIENCE

Advisory Editor
GERALD N. GROB

Editorial Board
ERIC T. CARLSON
BLANCHE D. COLL
CHARLES E. ROSENBERG

Recollections of
RICHARD DEWEY
Pioneer in
American Psychiatry

ARNO PRESS
A NEW YORK TIMES COMPANY
New York • 1973

Reprint Edition 1973 by Arno Press Inc.

Reprinted from a copy in
 The University of Illinois Library

MENTAL ILLNESS AND SOCIAL POLICY:
 The American Experience
ISBN for complete set: 0-405-05190-5
See last pages of this volume for titles.

Manufactured in the United States of America

———————◆———————

Library of Congress Cataloging in Publication Data

Dewey, Richard Smith, 1845-1933.
   Recollections of Richard Dewey.

   (Mental illness and social policy: the American
experience)
   Reprint of the ed. published by The University of
Cnicago Press, Chicago.
   Bibliography: p.
   √1.   Dewey, Richard Smith, 1845-1933.   I.   Title.
II.   Series.   [DNLM: l.   Psychiatry--History.   WZ100
D519?r 1936F]
RC339.52.D49A33 1973   616.8'9'00924 [B]   73-2395
ISBN 0-405-05203-0

Recollections of

RICHARD DEWEY

THE UNIVERSITY OF CHICAGO PRESS, CHICAGO

THE BAKER & TAYLOR COMPANY, NEW YORK; THE CAMBRIDGE UNIVERSITY
PRESS, LONDON; THE MARUZEN-KABUSHIKI-KAISHA, TOKYO, OSAKA,
KYOTO, FUKUOKA, SENDAI; THE COMMERCIAL PRESS, LIMITED, SHANGHAI

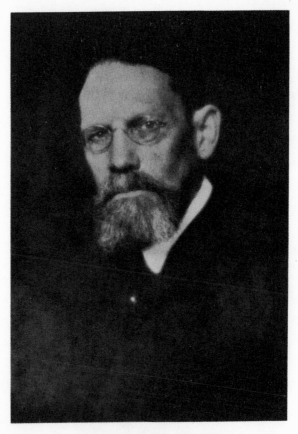

RICHARD DEWEY IN 1900

Recollections of
RICHARD DEWEY
Pioneer in
American Psychiatry

An Unfinished Autobiography
with an Introduction by
CLARENCE B. FARRAR, M.D.
Editor, *American Journal of Psychiatry*

Edited by ETHEL L. DEWEY

THE UNIVERSITY OF CHICAGO PRESS
CHICAGO · ILLINOIS

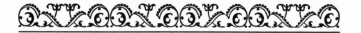

EDITOR'S NOTE

THE life of the author of these *Recollections* covered a period of more than fourscore years—from 1845 in New York State, when Indians still roamed its forests and the beginnings of the American railways were made, to 1933. He saw America develop from covered wagon to airplane. He had planned to give in the third part of the book an account of his more than fifty years of active practice in psychiatry, of his experience in his profession in its many aspects—scientific, social, legal, and administrative. He had completed the account of but twenty of those years at the time of his death.

The editor wishes to express her grateful appreciation for assistance and advice in the publication of this volume to Professor Sophonisba P. Breckinridge and Dean Edith Abbott, of the School of Social Service Administration, the University of Chicago; to Dr. G. Alder Blumer; Dr. Peter Bassoe; Ellinor M. Dewey; and to Dr. Clarence B. Farrar, writer of the Introduction.

INTRODUCTION

I T IS a privilege to say a word by way of introduction to the autobiography of Richard Dewey, whose death in 1933 removed a distinguished physician and a pioneer and leader in the modern period of American psychiatry.

This epoch is significant not merely for the student of medical history because of the striking changes in the concept of mental illness and the reforms and advances which have been achieved in methods of treatment; it is momentous for the observer of social movements in a larger sense as gauged by the attitude of society and of the state to the mental patient, and by the provisions made for his care.

When Dr. Dewey entered upon his psychiatric career, indiscriminate herding would be the words fairly to characterize the living conditions of the mentally ill in public institutions almost everywhere. To him is due the credit of introducing the method of segregation known as the "cottage plan," whereby the population of a large institution may be housed in small groups in separate buildings in order to secure the advantages and eliminate as far as possible the disadvantages of community life and thus facilitate treatment. This step, taken in 1879, when he assumed duty as the first superintendent of the new state hospital in Kankakee, Illinois, was Dr. Dewey's first great contribution to psychiatry. He had no precedent to follow in planning the administration of the new type of hospital; and the significance of the innovation may be realized when it is recalled that in the accelerated building-programs throughout the country during the sixties and seventies, following the Civil War, provision was scarcely contemplated for separating even the acute or recoverable from the chronic cases. It was necessary to combat the opinion-inertia of those who, as Dr. Dewey tells us, "averred that it was a vicious principle to separate the insane into curable and incurable classes."

The Kankakee example was quickly followed in other states, and a half-century's experience since those pioneer days has confirmed the judgment of Dr. Dewey and those who worked with him, particularly Mr. Frederick H. Wines, secretary of the State Board of Charities.

In 1893 occurred one of those unsavory events which should make the overzealous partisans of state medicine pause and ponder. In that year

John P. Altgeld became governor of Illinois, the first Democratic governor since the Civil War. The privileges of patronage were his first concern, an abuse of which there have been too many examples unto the present day. The governing boards of all the state institutions were removed; new boards were appointed; and the resignations of state hospital superintendents, including Dr. Dewey, were called for. By this political fiat the state deprived itself of the services of one of its ablest administrators and a great humanitarian reformer. As Dr. E. N. Brush, writing of Dr. Dewey's career, has put it: "This action of Governor Altgeld ushered in a partisan control of the state hospitals of Illinois, from which they have never fully recovered."

Dr. Dewey's autobiography covers the events of a fascinatingly varied and busy life up to the time when he severed his connection with the state hospital service in 1893. Although he left notes dealing with his subsequent professional activities, which did not terminate until 1920, when he was seventy-five years old, and which reflected contemporary movements and developments in the fields of psychiatry and mental hygiene, it has been deemed more fitting to leave the manuscript as he left it than to complete it by an alien hand.

In 1895 Dr. Dewey became medical director

of the reorganized Milwaukee Sanitarium at Wauwatosa, Wisconsin, of which he remained the guiding genius for twenty-five years, instituting new methods and creating at Wauwatosa a standard of sanitarium therapy which made it a model institution of its kind to which patients flocked from far and near. Possibly he felt that these were his happiest and most fruitful years. He was the friend of every patient, and every patient was his friend. It may be questioned if any physician has been better loved by his patients than he, or revered by a wider circle of those to whom in line of duty he ministered.

Among the literary activities of Dr. Dewey should be mentioned his period (1894–97) as editor of the *American Journal of Insanity* (now the *American Journal of Psychiatry*), the official organ of the venerable American Medico-Psychological Association (now the American Psychiatric Association); also, his collaboration with five other leading American and Canadian psychiatrists—Henry M. Hurd, William F. Drewry, Charles W. Pilgrim, G. Alder Blumer, and T. J. W. Burgess—in the production of the monumental four-volume history, *The Institutional Care of the Insane in the United States and Canada*, which was published in 1916–17.

After his retirement from the directorship of the Milwaukee Sanitarium, Dr. Dewey turned to the western coast to spend his sunset years. There in his study in La Cañada, looking out upon the mountains and the inspiring California scene, he took stock of the rich years of his life; there he wrote these *Recollections*.

"Biography exists," writes Sir Sidney Lee, "to satisfy a natural instinct in man—the commemorative instinct—the universal desire to keep alive the memories of those who by character and exploits have distinguished themselves from the mass of mankind." Dr. Dewey was the most modest of men, as the style of his narrative attests; and yet the plain story, which was not without its colorful chapters, and all set forth so simply, likewise attests the character of the man and affords glimpses of the exploits which distinguished him.

His nature was a happy blending of courage and gentleness, of the philanthropic spirit and innate modesty, of humor and philosophy, of scientific thoroughness and artistic sensibility, and all his dealings instinct with the selflessness of the true gentleman. From his college days onward he has been a writer of songs and a maker of verse, and his wholesome boyishness disputed the claims of age to the last. In 1929 he suffered a severe illness, a pyloric perforation, necessitating an emergency operation. He was in his eighty-fourth year. His remarkable recovery was surely not due alone to physical strength and the skill of the surgeon, Dr. Leroy B. Sherry, of Pasadena; a youthful spirit and a will to health must also be reckoned with. If proof be needed, witness the following lines written by the convalescent patient. They afford a lesson in applied mental hygiene worth commemorating.

MEDITATION OF A GASTRO-ENTEROSTOMISÉ

Not long ago old Father Time and I
Again looked one another in the eye.
Quoth he: "You now have passed your eighty-third;
You seem to be a rather tough old bird;
From me you can expect but little more;
Behave yourself and even up the score.
I gave you a pyloric perforation—
Don't think that you deserve the least laudation
Because you have survived the operation—
The surgeon's skill and pluck were your salvation."

Then I resentfully and proudly spoke:
"A gastro-enterostomy's no joke;
Yet, thanks, I'm feeling now quite merry—
Despite dry law I had some shots of Sherry."

And so without more ado we turn the page, and Richard Dewey speaks for himself.

C. B. F.

CONTENTS

I

EARLY YEARS; SCHOOL; COLLEGE

II

EXPERIENCES OF AN AMERICAN VOLUNTEER ASSISTANT SURGEON IN THE FRANCO-PRUSSIAN WAR

III

THE YEARS 1871–1893

ILLINOIS HOSPITALS FOR THE INSANE; ORIGIN AND GROWTH OF THE INSTITUTION AT KANKAKEE, ILLINOIS; EARLY PSYCHIATRISTS

TITLES OF PAPERS BY RICHARD DEWEY

INDEX

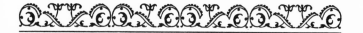

CHAPTER ONE

Early Years; School; College

I WAS BORN on December 6, 1845, at Forestville, Chautauqua County, New York, a son of the village blacksmith and gristmill-owner, Elijah Dewey, whose father, Elijah Dewey, Sr., had fought in the Revolutionary War. We were descended from Thomas Dewey, of Sandwich, Kent, England, who landed in 1633 at Dorchester, Massachusetts. My mother was Sophia Smith, daughter of Richard Smith (born in Danby, Vermont, in 1780), who settled in Hamburg, Erie County, New York. He was a justice of the peace and member of the New York State assembly in 1816 and 1817.

Chautauqua County is the westernmost county of the Empire State, and is famed for the altitude of Chautauqua Lake, thirteen hundred feet above sea-level, "opening an eye to heaven"; and also for the Chautauqua Institute, founded by Bishop Vincent, a nation-wide influence in popular and religious education, the "alma mater" of many Chautauqua circles throughout the nation. Near at hand are the Great Lakes, Erie and Ontario, and Niagara River connecting them, with the stupendous cataract between. These wonders are famous, but Chautauqua's little village of Forestville has never drawn attention from the outside world. It was and is a village of a few hundred souls, five miles from Lake Erie, which grew up on the banks of Walnut Creek, the creek being named no doubt from the great black-walnut tree that overshadowed its banks at that point. The story of the great tree will come later in my narrative; I must here recount an escape from drowning that occurred in my third year, the earliest event in my remembrance. That escape, and the others of my eighty-five years, make possible this adding of one more to the autobiographies of the day; it is the earliest picture that impressed me, and remains vivid today. An older brother, Henry, was sitting by the cistern feeding chickens. I sat down beside him and, when told to look out lest I fall in, said that I "guessed" I could sit there as well as he. Hardly had this boastful utterance been delivered when I toppled over. A shout from one or both of us called the "hired girl," Maria Doolittle, who happened to be near. She was a paragon of faithfulness and presence of mind; I see her as plainly today as I did then, reaching for me, grasping my gingham

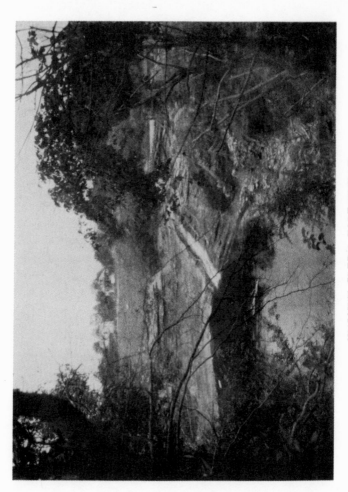

WALNUT CREEK, FORESTVILLE

dress, and lifting me out all dripping before I had time to realize my danger.

The landscape of boyhood has a background of hill and forest, but the foreground is occupied by Walnut Creek (we pronounced it *crik*). It may be that geographers take little note of Walnut Creek; it was, nevertheless, an important stream to the boys of Forestville. Therein these village urchins were wont to swim in summer, and thereon to skate in winter, while therefrom at various seasons they gleefully drew forth the silvery "shiner," the bristling "pumpkin-seed," the chubby "red-horn dace," not to mention the "sucker," less esteemed. We found these finny fellows as interesting as the more ambitious anglers of today find the speckled or rainbow trout, the pike or pickerel. There was one lad of my acquaintance who, having a strong belief in the efficacy of prayer, when casting forth his line, having duly spat upon the wriggling bait, would tightly shut his eyes and repeat some sentences of the Pater Noster. He would end: "Thy will be done," in earnest expectation of results, leaving to overruling providence the reward for his act of faith. The outcome of his system, however, was not such as to encourage its continuance. There were various customs known to the boys of those days; I wonder if they are still observed. Do boys still spit on the bait when fishing? If they still play "one ole cat," do they moisten the palm for a good grip upon the bat? When making ready to "rassle" ("side holt" or "square holt"), do they expectorate upon the palm with that mixture of superstition and practicality?

Aside from fishing, Walnut Creek had other allurements; there was the drop it took over the great ledge of rock into the "Deep Hole." There stood my father's blacksmith shop, gristmill, the millpond and dam, and behind the mill the deep swimming-hole, a natural basin, where the men and boys could disport themselves. On the high bank at one side was the diving-place, whence the brave could plunge into the depths below. On the other side were shallows, safe for beginners. From this rustic natatorium, Walnut Creek meandered onward in rocky gorge, reaching a still-water basin, with rock bottom, not over one's head, and shut in on both sides by shelving walls and forest trees—a secluded bathing pool where at times the girls were allowed to swim. Here was a grapevine swing; thick twisted ropes of wild grape hanging from the trees above made a wonderful trapeze. In the walls of the gorge were caverns and recesses where a boy bandit could conceal himself with his plunder. The more adventurous indulged at night in games of "Hi, spy," one party pursuing another from hiding-place to hiding-place, full of the zest of chase and capture. I remember the regret I suffered when a solicitous mother forbade my joining these marauders.

The millpond was at the foot of Sheridan Hill, to me a mighty eminence, in reality measuring nearly a half-mile from base to summit. There in winter we went to coast (we called it "sliding down hill"). This hill, when covered with snow, was a perfect toboggan slide, steep and varied with "thank-you-ma'ams"; down this slope the adventurous boy, coming "belly blunt" on his sled to its foot, had only to turn a little to the left to slide on over the bank of the Creek, out on the smooth surface of the millpond, gliding, if he had skill, to the very brink of the milldam.

In those winters of the eighteen-forties and fifties, such snowstorms occurred as, if memory can be trusted, are not known today. Sheridan Hill would perhaps seem less precipitous to the adult, but one thing is certain: we built snowhouses in the drifts on this hill in which a grown man could stand erect, because a grown man did —a big brother five feet eight inches in height. Those snowhouses aroused more interest and gave more delight than could marble palaces today.

Among the stories arousing wonder which were known to every child in Forestville was the story of the great hollow walnut tree that had been lived in as a house; had served as a wayside inn;

had finally been taken down and floated on the lake to Buffalo; sailed next on the Erie Canal to Albany; then down the Hudson to New York. From there, after being exhibited to thousands, it had been taken to London and shown in a museum. This great tree stood on the bank of Walnut Creek, half on the village highway, half upon our gristmill property. It had blown down in April, 1822, and lay for a long time where it fell.[1] Finally in 1825 it occurred to a citizen who operated a grocery store near by to make practical use of the prostrate giant. The roots and upper branches were cut away, leaving a section of the trunk thirteen feet high and thirty-one feet in circumference; this, when hollowed out, formed a shell whose wall was four inches thick. Four yokes of oxen and the labor of twelve men had been required to accomplish this. As the trunk lay on its side, a man on horseback, with head bent to the horse's neck, was able to ride through the trunk. It was now placed in an upright position; and a door hung with strap hinges was contrived, also a floor and roof. The grocer had a circular plank seat built around the inside of his "Tree Tavern" and a table placed in the center. Hereon various kinds of liquor were set

[1] The details of the story of this tree are taken from the "Seventh Paper of the Hanover History" by G. L. Heaton, published in the *Fredonia Censor* (New York) and reprinted in the *Silver Creek News* (New York), June 26, 1924.

forth; and many travelers (twenty or more a day), some on their way west in covered wagons, stopped for rest and refreshment. The proprietor, however, had an experience which made of him an ultra total abstainer such as was seldom known in that early day: some Indians from the neighboring Catteraugus Reservation got so drunk on his liquor that, while camping around a fire near by that night, one of them in his drunken sleep rolled into the fire and was horribly burned. For several weeks he was a pitiable, helpless mass of corruption; the keeper of the Tree Tavern took care of him and vowed he would never again sell to anybody, or drink, a drop of intoxicating liquor.

The tree had not long done service for the tavern-owner before others aspired to possess it. After considerable negotiation two men, dwellers in the vicinity, gained control and engaged in a plan for the exploitation of what remained of the forest giant. The new owners at once began making plans for getting the tree to Buffalo. A merchant of Dunkirk, owner of a small schooner, agreed to tow the shell down Silver Creek to Lake Erie. To accomplish the haul to Silver Creek they had a truck constructed, making the wheels from the largest maple logs to be found. The truck was completed and the shell loaded upon it one Saturday noon (the schooner lying at anchor at the mouth of Silver Creek). Two strings of five yokes of oxen each were hitched to the trucks, but in the first start the reach gave way and the forward trucks slid from under the load. After a delay for repair, early on Sunday morning they made a new start, this time with success; the ten yokes of oxen hauled the huge trunk through the main street of Forestville. Heaton, then a boy of five, remembered being called at dawn to take a last look at what remained of the great black walnut as it passed his father's door. Borne next by schooner and Lake Erie vessel, the tree reached Buffalo. The proprietors exhibited it with but poor success, failing to make expenses. The next spring there were new owners, who, as soon as the Erie Canal opened, made preparations to take the tree to New York. Since no canal boat could float its great bulk under the bridges on the way, the tree was sawed in two and the parts loaded on an open canal boat. In New York (the parts having been skilfully riveted together) the tree drew immense crowds, and the receipts were far greater than could have been predicted. In 1827 it was sold for two thousand dollars to a London purchaser. Finally it was destroyed by fire in a London museum whose owner had knocked out part of his wall to get it under cover. So ends the story of the Big Black Walnut of Chautauqua County.

The places and people of the hamlet of Forestville live in my memory today. The dwellers upon its streets, lanes, and roadways were interesting people to the curiosity of a boy. But if a
hamlet, as Forestville was called, is "a cluster of
buildings without a church," the word does not
apply, for we had both Baptist and Methodist
houses of worship. The latter stood upon the village green near the schoolhouse and playground,
where at recess we played the games of prison
goal, "cangalo," crack-the-whip, bull-in-the-ring,
and ball games of various types. The Methodist
church had a platform along its front, at one end
quite high above the ground. Here we competed
at flying jump, running the length of the platform to spring from the high end; and with con-
ceit of pardonable pride the writer records, or
admits, that he was holder of the record for the
flying jump; his were the heels which left a mark
in the earth no other boy in the "Little Room"
could overpass. (Our school did not have grades;
it had but two divisions: the Little Room and
the Big Room.)

The shallow pond in Walnut Creek above the
mill was the scene on an occasional Sunday of a
religious ceremony which always brought a con-
course of spectators—the baptism by immersion
of converts secured during the periodical reviv-
als. Sometimes the event took place in winter,

and a parallelogram of large dimensions had to be cut in the ice to make possible the required complete immersion. We found it exciting to see the minister and the disciples in their black robes wade into the ice-cold stream, especially if a nervous lady were the subject of the ceremony and if she came up sputtering and gasping after being "dipped." Certain of the adherents to this church were called "free-will Baptists," while others were of the "hard-shell" variety; but the distinction was never fully grasped by the boy spectators.

Some of the dwellers in our village were interesting people. There was the Caledonian clan: three brothers, with their families, who had come from Scotland. One was named James, a landed proprietor, a kindly man who spoke with a pleasant burr and sang Scotch songs with spirit. He had large hayfields; and I remember one year when, just as he had got in a great crop of hay, his barn was struck by lightning, and barn and hay went up in smoke. It was then recalled that he had kept his men at work on Sunday, and certain of the orthodox were convinced that the fire was a judgment upon the Sabbath-breaker. The second of the brothers was a doctor; the Scotch highball had not then been heard of, but the doctor took his scotch straight, and often in such liberal drafts that he was visibly half-seas over. The townspeople were divided in their opinion of him: if it were not for drink, some said, he would be at the head of his profession; others held that he was better when intoxicated than any sober doctor for miles around. The third Caledonian brother gave the town a great shock by ending his own existence in an attack of delirium.

The advent of the Episcopal church, hitherto unknown in the town, was an event of interest. The Episcopal bishop had occasionally visited and conducted service; his robes, with lawn sleeves "as big as a bag of wheat," were impressive to people of plain Puritan antecedents. After a time, a little Episcopalian chapel stood upon the green, where schoolhouse and Methodist and Baptist churches had dominated. The service of the new church, with its chants, its "getting up and sitting down," and short sermon, was a great contrast to the services we had known; it gave a solemnity to the new, small chapel. My parents were of the Presbyterian faith, but their church was five miles away and they could not attend regularly. It happened that my sister and I were asked to lead the singing in the new chapel; carrying the treble, I learned thus to chant the psalms of David to the accompaniment of the melodeon under my sister's hands. A pipe organ of modest dimensions had been part of our household furniture; and after a time when a new, and as it seemed to us, *grand* new Methodist church was built, and the acquiring of an organ was under consideration, this instrument of ours was purchased and installed in the new church. As a result of the transfer, we obtained a pianoforte (called "pianoforty" by the boys). There was one other such in the entire village, an instrument of magic and wonder. Upon its arrival my friends gathered and perched on the fence in front of the house to hear it played. Vocal music of a primitive kind was common in those days; and the "singing school" was an important feature of the winter season, promoting both song and sociability. On Sunday afternoons the "family sing," of exclusively religious songs, was a customary event; "Rock of Ages," "Joy to the World, the Lord Is Come," and "From Greenland's Icy Mountains" were some of the favorites. On weekdays, however, there was a great variety; and strains and snatches of ballads and ditties were heard wherever the people assembled. "A Little More Cider," "Jordan Am a Hard Road," "Old Uncle Ned," were known to all. There were songs of sentiment, too, sung by sweet-voiced girls: "Blue Juanita," "Bounding Billows," and "Highland Mary."

One boyhood companion I would mention here had a large share of my affection—Joe Adams, son of an Irish farm laborer, a clever and good-

hearted boy, possessed of unusual natural gifts.
He could locate the ground-birds' and bank-
swallows' nests; could point out in the trees where
the robins and orioles had built; could collect the
eggs; knew the ways of birds with their young;
and knew the best places to gather berries in
summer and chestnuts in fall. He knew the customs of bees, which ones would sting; also, certain whitefaced ones that could be handled with
impunity. He would wait half an hour for my
lesson to end so that we might go to the woods
together.

Our home was in the strict Puritan tradition:
family prayers, grace at table; seven Bible verses
must be learned every Saturday for Sunday
school; the shorter catechism and the Ten Com-
mandments must be memorized. A gentle but
earnest mother so winningly urged these tasks
that the irksomeness was scarcely felt. The books
in the house were few—*History of the Reforma-
tion*, Baxter's *Saint's Rest*, *Pilgrim's Progress*,
Barnes's *Notes on the New Testament*. When I was
seven, *Uncle Tom's Cabin* came into the house,
the first fiction I had known. *The Arabian
Nights*, and *Robinson Crusoe* came in due time,
though there was a serious question regarding the
Thousand and One Nights. About this time my
older brother began to read Robert Bonner's *New
York Ledger* and the so-called "blood-and-thun-

der" serials. My curiosity was piqued by these highly seasoned tales, which brought the world of crime and violence for the first time to my mind. On dark nights I now hurried home, imagining possible points of ambush beset with kidnapers and robbers.

At this time there came to the family circle a granduncle who had experiences to relate on two strikingly attractive subjects: the Revolutionary War and spiritualism. During the war, Granduncle Gray, as a boy of thirteen, had been ordered to sentinel duty on a wooded border. At night, alone, he shouldered his musket and patrolled his beat. What sounded like a heavy tread and then a loud report startled the young sentinel out of ability to control his cowardly legs. He fled, ostensibly to report the incursion of the enemy; and, returning with reinforcements, he discovered that a calf had likewise been patrolling the wood. Granduncle Gray had attended seances, then first known through the Fox Sisters, who had developed revelations of spirit life by means of "spirit rappings." A son of his, a New York homeopathic physician, famous and successful in his day, had lost a beloved wife and hoped for a message from the "spirit land." Seances had been held in his house, at which my granduncle told of having seen musical instruments floating in the air, giving out music; of having heard bells rung

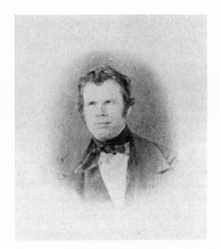

ELIJAH DEWEY

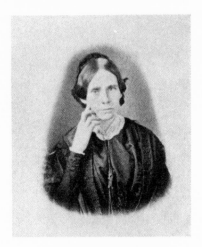

SOPHIA SMITH DEWEY

by invisible means. He aroused our open-mouthed wonder.

The first influx of Irish and German immigrants became known to me as a school boy in the late forties, when the New York and Erie Railroad was being pushed through Forestville to Dunkirk, its terminus on Lake Erie. Irish track laborers were encamped along the right of way, and German and Irish families began to settle in our midst. The ways and speech of these new-comers attracted our attention, and we were not free from a sense of superiority in contemplating them; we called them "outlandish," which to us meant inferior. Still, though we condescended, we were not unfriendly; it was in a spirit of play that we called the German school fellow "nix kom 'raus." There was one Pat who, being found still much exhilarated on the day after the Fourth of July, said he was "celebratin' the Fifth." When he was given a blanket, shown to the freight house, and advised to "sleep it off," he complied and, before dropping off, said a prayer, invoking a blessing upon certain benefactors, one of whom was Elijah Dewey, my father. Mention of the Fourth calls to my mind one of the great occasions of the year, the "General Training" on that day, the outstanding feature of which was the parade of the "fusileers," a burlesque procession of rustics, mock soldiers on horseback, in fantastic uniforms, with flintlock guns, antique swords, and cocked hats.

When the New York and Erie Railroad was nearing completion in the winter of 1850–51, I rode in a sleigh to the bridge over the "deep cut" near our ten-acre lot, and witnessed beneath the bridge the iron horse snortingly chugging and plowing over the snow-covered track, pulling freight baggage and passengers to their destination. It was my first view of a steam locomotive, the marvel of the day. The following summer, when the road was in working order, a celebration occurred. People came from far and near; Daniel Webster was present as orator of the occasion. There was a barbecue—a whole ox roasted in a pit; the multitudes ate and drank. To my sorrow, I knew of these events only from hearing them described (and was no doubt the more vividly impressed) because I was held to be too young to take part, and had to stay at home.

The echoes of a stirring world-event reached our village in 1852, when Louis Kossuth came to the United States to plead for Hungary, then languishing under Austrian tyranny. From one end of the country to the other his eloquent voice was heard. The emblem of the event to me, at seven, was a Kossuth hat, with black ostrich feather, which I proudly wore.

There occurred in those years many contacts

with our native Indians. Indian foot races and lacrosse games were a feature of the Chautauqua County Fair; no white man could compete with the red in endurance and speed. The Cattaraugus Reservation had been established near us, and there a mission sought to win the Indian to the white man's ways of life, of farming, and of religion. We frequently visited the Reservation, and saw many who lived, in their native manner, almost wholly by hunting and fishing. A troupe of Indians in their grotesque feathers and war paint held an exhibition in our village. They went through the motions of capturing and scalping their victims, and gave their blood-curdling war whoop, "eee—yah," which we tried vainly to imitate.

Across Walnut Creek from the village center, close by the bridge, stood the blacksmith shop and the dwelling of my father. We had a few acres which provided a garden and plenty of play space. Our boundaries were the main street on one side and Walnut Creek on the west and south. In those days homeopathy and hydropathy were coming to be known as a reaction against the older and more drastic methods of the allopathic school. A doctor of the new school, who desired to establish a water cure, offered nineteen hundred dollars for our home, with its frontage on the Creek, and other buildings suitable for his purpose. The sale was completed; and while the new house was building, we lived in a temporary home across the creek. Our family doctor, though of the old school, was tolerant of the new cult. Before long, a medical establishment replaced our former home, and included a bath house on the bank of the creek. I remember the names of the new medicines: pulsatilla; aconite, and belladonna. A drop of each in a glass of water, a teaspoonful from each glass given alternately an hour apart, served as a specific for many a childish ailment.

My father before long was owner of the gristmill below the smithy on Walnut Creek. He had saved enough to enable him to build a new house on the building-site opposite our former home. There in due time we inhabited a cottage upon the little plateau overlooking the mill and garden and the buildings below. There was, on the higher level, the grateful shade of some old apple trees; and the modest white house with its green blinds was a happy home to the children for many a year and a hospitable stopping-place to many a wayfarer, colporteur, and traveling "missioner." Adjoining the new house was the dwelling of the head miller, an ancient craftsman who knew the arts of grinding grains both coarse and fine—provender for cows and pigs, "snowflake" for the housewife. Across the transverse street was the family-doctor's home, the good doctor whose vines and trees produced such delicious grapes and cherries. Here I learned the lesson of forbidden fruit and found there is such a thing in the world as *meum et teum*, for I was apprehended in the grape arbor by the doctor himself one bright Sunday morning, in the act of stuffing mouth and pockets with luscious Concords. Young boys may be unconscious of guilt in the appropriation of others' goods; but my sense of guilt was overpowering when, in the Sunday school the same morning, the doctor, who was also superintendent, addressing the assembled classes, enlarged upon the sins of larceny, grand and petty. I trembled in anticipation of being held up before the school as a terrible example. The painful moments passed, however, with denunciation of the crime, the criminal being left to the stings of conscience, which were all too soon forgotten. This, moreover, was a second offense; at an earlier time I had taken from my uncle's hardware store a tin flageolet and, after escaping with the booty, while speculating upon the possible consequences of such crime, had asked an older brother whether the raptor of a tin whistle could be sent to the state prison.

Primitive was the life of those days. The fine arts, as we esteem them, were unknown; yet was there charm and allurement all about us. The love of beauty would not be denied. Painted landscapes had we none; yet we were content with nature's fields, woods, and streams. Daguerre had made his great invention and gave us rare likeness of form and feature. The movable studio, that came as a wheeled vehicle to our town, waited on the public green for all who cared to "sit for a portrait." In this studio-on-wheels were produced daguerreotypes that gave back our countenances with seeming magic; to my own eyes I looked quite alive in my steel-buttoned gray-velvet jacket; and my gentle mother and sister in sober raiment showed spiritual light and life in face, form, and feature.

Every year when late autumn came, the gathering of nuts made the Saturday business and pleasure of many a boy. What could be more alluring than the ripening treasures of these splendid nut trees? Picnicking was combined with the pleasure of accumulating a winter's store of these delicious edibles, to be consumed in chestnut roasts, candy-pulls, and corn-popping festivities in the winter evenings. Spring, too, had its special joys. Before the snow had melted, numerous "sugar bushes"—tracts of maple-sugar trees—were tapped for the abundance of their sweet sap, which, when boiled, made syrup and cakes of maple sugar. Farmers coming to mill brought quantities of maple sugar, which my father took for home consumption. Keen was our delight when the boiling-time arrived; then we made parties for the "sugaring-off." This took place when the syrup was at the right stage for making maple honey. Snow was spread in pans, and the syrup poured upon it. The patties thus created surpassed, in richness and flavor, the confectioner's finest bon bons.

Here let me record some impressions, imbibed in my sixth to tenth years, of the crafts of the blacksmith and miller. My father, when he started out in life, was the village blacksmith; later he was owner of the gristmill. The smithy stood on the bank of Walnut Creek, where he owned some acres. The words of Longfellow's poem were true of him: "a mighty man was he"; he, too, "owed no man anything"; and he, too, "heard his daughter singing in the village choir." Well I remember how children, coming home from school, looked in at the open smithy door. Many times I stood when the smith was at work, blowing the bellows till the fire glowed, and then, with his tongs taking out the white-hot iron, shaping it with hammer blows upon his anvil, into horseshoes, spikes, rings, bolts, lynch pins, implements of many sorts. He would rapidly turn a slender iron rod into horseshoe nails, with tapering points and polygonal heads. The glow of the flying sparks and the roar of the bellows were an accompaniment to the ring of the hammer blows on the anvil. When a horse was to be shod, the smith would take between his knees upon his leather apron the light or clumsy shank, holding it firmly until the restive animal was quiet, then trim and pare the horny hoof, nail on the nicely fitted shoe, deftly driving home each nail; would turn and clip the projecting points; then make all smooth with the rasp. Runners for a sleigh, tires for cart or buggy wheel, skates for a boy—all were shaped on his anvil.

I came to know the mill even better than the smithy. Let me try to picture it: The mill stood upon the great ledge of rock at the top of which the dam held back the waters of the millpond, guiding them into the flume beneath the mill where the reserve waters lay in readiness to be launched upon the waiting mill wheel whenever the miller should lift the gates. When the gates were lifted, the water coursed from the flume over the great overshot wheel, dropping some twenty feet in turning it and, at the lower level, racing out into the big swimming-hole at the base of the falls. The front elevation of the mill was two stories in height; but, extending backward, as it did, over the precipitous rock ledge, five stories were required to bring the rear to a height level with the front. Before the entrance ran the platform where the farmers unloaded their wheat,

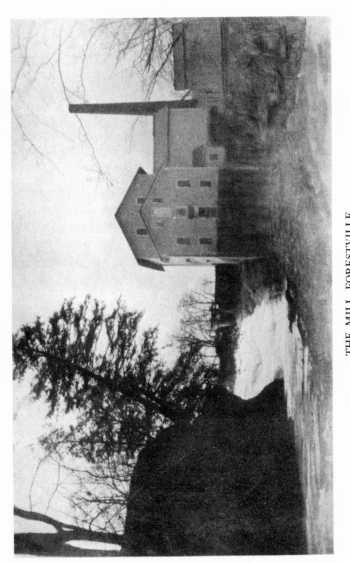

THE MILL, FORESTVILLE

corn, and oats. Here the miller and the arriving
rustics exchanged greetings. One standing pleas-
antry between them went as follows: "Well, what
do ye know?" "I know the miller has fat pigs."
Then the miller would reply: "Is there anything
you don't know?" "Yes—whose grain they're
eating."

The shaft of the great wheel propelled the cogs
and pinions which operated the three ponderous
pairs of millstones, the nether bedded in con-
crete, while the upper revolved inexorably, crush-
ing the hard kernels into flour or meal as they
fell from the hopper. The whole wheat flour was
conveyed to the revolving sieves, made of finest
bolting-cloth. These sieves deposited the snowy
drifts in bags and barrels below; and at the end
of the sifting, the middlings, shorts, and bran fell
out (these could not pass the sieves). This coarser
stuff was called canaille (canell); at a later time
it took high rank as healthful graham flour and
bran. From it then was made "emptyings," used
universally in place of yeast, to raise the salt-
rising bread, the only kind we knew. Flour was
sometimes brought back to the mill, with the
complaint of some good housewife that it did not
make white-enough bread. Then loaves which
could not be excelled for whiteness would be
made in the miller's kitchen, to test whether the
fault was in the flour. One delicious product of

the mill which we enjoyed in the late fall was samp. It was made from corn which was just ripe enough to be coarsely ground and which made a cereal the like of which I have never seen or tasted since. One who had enjoyed this delicious flavor could not forget it. Another delicacy we often enjoyed was parched corn, partially baked in the oven, ground in the coffee mill, and eaten with cream and sugar. One more product of the mill I would name—provender for cattle, which was made by putting corn on the cob through the corn-cracker and then letting the millstones grind it.

Once my father came upon me in the mill, loitering, as he supposed, and playing with one of the pinion jacks. It had slipped, and the miller had asked me to hold it while he went below to make repairs. My father thought I was meddling, and gave me a little cuff. When he found I was not at fault, he made amends. I always remembered this apology, made to me, a child. A kindly father was he. Once when, for inexcusable delay, he had intimated a reckoning was due me, it was never made. Whether he forgot, or purposely let me go unpunished, I never knew. Unlike her husband, my mother was not too soft-hearted to inflict condign but prayerful punishment upon a careless or disobedient boy. Dust was an unavoidable accompaniment of mill life, and the dusty miller was occasionally brushed off good-naturedly by the vigilant housewife; she was an inveterate enemy of dust, but always lenient toward my father on these occasions.

An important event at the mill was the sharpening of the millstones—a process the machine age knows not of; can barely recall. It involved cessation of grinding for a time, when a strange silence, followed by unwonted sounds, took possession of the mill. The massive upper stone was lifted by a crane and swung to one side; then, with steel picks tempered to the utmost hardness, the upper and under surfaces of the flinty "French burr" stones were gone over, fretting the grinding ridges with fine parallel cuts. Thus the stones were periodically sharpened anew for their work. The making and tempering of the picks was an exacting job. The blacksmith heated them in the forge and sharpened them to the keenest cutting edge, then plunged them at the right moment into the tempering tub, to give a hardness of adamant.

The contrast between the primitive time of which I write and the present day in respect to domestic economy and home industries is very striking. It was only for exceptional things that we went outside the home. Our chickens, cows, calves, sheep, and pigs produced the food we required, including fresh meat and cured. The garden and orchard gave abundant vegetables and fruits, fresh in season, pickled and preserved for winter. Soap and candles were made at home, though kerosene soon replaced candles. And what of bread, the staff of life? The wheat, of course, came from a neighbor's farm; and the flour, from the mill instead of from the grocery as now; and every home produced its own daily bread, mostly "salt-raised," also its pastry and cakes. Spinning was a common art, for the knitting of socks, mittens, and mufflers. Cotton and woolen cloth were mostly purchased; wares of the tailor and shoemaker were made in every village; frequently a woman tailor went from house to house.

There were no machines for mowing and reaping. The scythe is still known; not so the cradle for cutting grain or the flail for threshing it: the cradle was an attachment on the scythe which held the stalks until they were thrown in parallel rows on the ground, to be caught up and bound in sheaves or shocks. The flail consisted of two heavy sticks loosely tied together, end to end, by a leather thong, one stick used as a handle, the other made to pound or thresh the grain left on the barn floor when the straw had been removed.

The fall migration of innumerable flocks of pigeons was an exciting event. Though they have now disappeared, they flew south in every autumn of the fifties and sixties of the last century. Their migration gave rise to an undesirable industry, which explains why they are no longer seen. Men came with great nets, which they erected in the fields; stool pigeons were fastened to the ground as a lure. When the pigeons alighted, the nets fell upon them, trapping thousands for the city markets. The boys of Forestville, too, captured pigeons in a more decent manner, "pot-hunting"; their exploits were irreverently celebrated in the following quatrain, parodying a hymn of Isaac Watts:

> When I can shoot my rifle clear
> To pigeons in the sky,
> I'll bid farewell to pork and beans
> And live on pigeon pie.

During the years 1856–60, in my tenth to fourteenth years, the antislavery struggle was going on, and I was conscious of the echoes of the great conflict. My father had been a "Henry Clay Whig" since 1840, when this party triumphantly elected William Henry Harrison. That had been an exciting campaign, with its much-heard slogan, its rallies and processions. In the eighteen-fifties the new Republican party came into being; and in 1856 General Frémont, the explorer, "Pathfinder" of a way to the Pacific, was nominated for the presidency. The campaign slogan, "Free speech, free soil, and Frémont," was heard on every side; and Horace Greeley's *New York Tribune*, of which my father was a diligent reader, was the leading organ of the new party. There was an emotional and romantic interest in the campaign. What actually amounted to civil war was even then in progress in "bleeding Kansas," where slaveholders were attempting to force slavery upon a free state. The fugitive-slave decision of the Supreme Court, the operations of the Underground Railroad, the violent assault upon Charles Sumner in the United States Senate, the execution of John Brown in December, 1859, the Lincoln and Douglas senatorial debates—all these events aroused the interest and fighting spirit of old and young. I attended mass meetings and heard Governor Seward's oration on the "Irrepressible Conflict." On election day in 1856 I tied up bundles of ballots for my father, to be distributed by him at the polls. Mass meetings and political rallies varied the monotony of village life, and in 1860 came the Lincoln Wide-Awakes with torchlight processions.

In 1858, when I was twelve, occurred a momentous change for me, from quiet, rustic home life to the bustling halls, classrooms, and dormitories of a boarding-school. The older heads thought it wise for the youth to go to "college." I was myself conscious of some degree of ambition to study. To Dwight's Rural School, in Clinton,

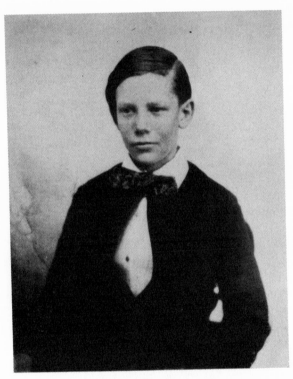

RICHARD DEWEY, YOUTH

New York, it was decided I should go. The preparation for entering the school seemed, in my case, to be chiefly sartorial. Of book knowledge outside that already inculcated in the "big" schoolroom, only a slight acquaintance with Latin was required. (I was to have, in Benjamin Dwight, an illustrious teacher of Latin and Greek); but the clothes to be worn in the new environment exacted much attention. In Forestville there were no clothing-stores; clothes of young boys were made at home by a "tailoress." A black roundabout of 1857 model had been provided me, which replaced a much regretted velvet jacket, "speckled like a trout," which had been my Sunday coat of previous years. Now the black roundabout was out of style and must be altered. A change in sleeves had been decreed: they must now be expanded at the wrist. So the good black sleeve was ripped, and Serepta Devine, the clubfooted tailoress, inserted a wedge or gusset. This wedge was later to become a cause of grief to me, and is indelibly fixed in my memory; other details of the outfit have faded from remembrance. On the day of departure for Clinton my mother sent me for a talk with my father, who wanted a parting word with me. That word was never fully spoken; as we two walked side by side, sentences began but were broken off unfinished. A deep emotion moved this father, who had himself known little schooling; he wanted to tell his son how keen were his hopes that he should be worthy of the expectations of those who loved him. In truth, though the exhortation found few words, it was not without response in the heart of the not-too-serious lad.

This was the first year of the school in its new location at Clinton. For twelve years it had been conducted at Brooklyn, New York, where more than two thousand young men had been drilled in its halls and classrooms; many had there been inspired to worthy careers. Benjamin Dwight was an educator of the noblest ideals and of unflagging zeal in their realization. He was himself a grandson of the illustrious first president of Yale, Timothy Dwight. He had graduated in arts at Hamilton and in divinity at Yale. He had now brought his school to the country, where he sought to make for the young men committed to his charge a home as well as a school, and to have a healthful environment for them, free from the disadvantages of the city. Here he could realize the aims he cherished: the boys were received into a home. The Rev. David A. Holbrook, an accomplished, able, and genial man was second in command and lived with his family in the school, creating the needed friendly atmosphere and fatherly oversight for the forty or fifty youths in residence. Here was made pos-

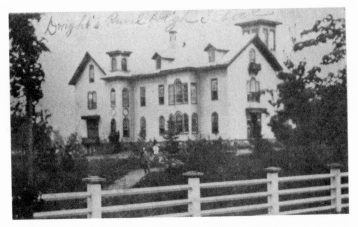

THE DWIGHT RURAL HIGH SCHOOL

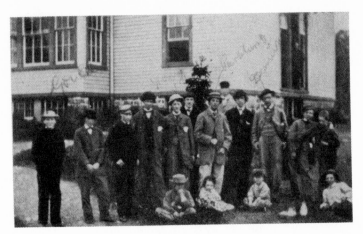

GROUP AT THE SCHOOL IN 1859

THE ORNAMENTATION THICK HEDGES.

GROUP AT THE FIRE, SCHOOL IN 1857.

sible a culture social, scholarly, and religious; physical training also was offered, which was unusual at that time. A spacious gymnasium had been constructed, equipped with the best apparatus then to be had; and Dr. Dio Lewis, a famous apostle of clean and healthful sport and "muscular Christianity," gave weekly talks and demonstrations; he had us rise early, sprint a half-mile or a mile before breakfast, take a cold shower, and advocated a training-table diet.

One of the distinguished attributes of Dr. Dwight was his eminence in the science and study of languages, ancient and modern. In addition to our classes in Latin, Greek, and mathematics, we were taught French and German, though in that day these languages were seldom in the curricula of either public or private schools. No one could be a pupil of Benjamin Dwight's without gaining a valuable insight into language and a broader appreciation of words, their origin and transformation; one learned of the development of language, traced from Sanskrit through Greek and Latin to modern forms.

Among the forty or fifty boys assembled in the Rural High School, there was a mingling of youths from country and city, twelve to twenty years of age; they came chiefly from New York and New England. To most, needless to say, games and fun were more interesting than books. We had the inevitable proportion of "Simps" and "Smart Alecs." I remember a boy who would give demonstrations of driving pins into his thigh, asserting it did not hurt him in the least. Another had a cure for warts: making a ball of cobweb, laying it on the wart, and setting it on fire, burning away wart and cobweb together. We were all ravenous for food; and on Saturdays we went to the woods and cooked oysters, eggs, and frogs' legs. It was in the year 1858 that baseball was first organized as played today; a diamond was laid out on our school grounds, with canvas bags to mark the bases. We played with the same ferocious energy that marks the game among school boys of today. In 1860 the school, as one man, was absorbed by interest in the great prize fight between Heenan, the California "Benicia Boy" and Tom Sayers, the English champion. Every incident of the fight was followed with the same intense interest that is shown in the contests of today; the sport page and camera, however, were absent from our world. We even had a pugilistic contest in the school, in which two of our boys fought to a decision with bare fists. The match was carried out with the crude rules then in force, prior to the adoption of the Marquis of Queensbury regulations.

A copy of Shakespeare was given me at the school; I found it so absorbing in interest that I

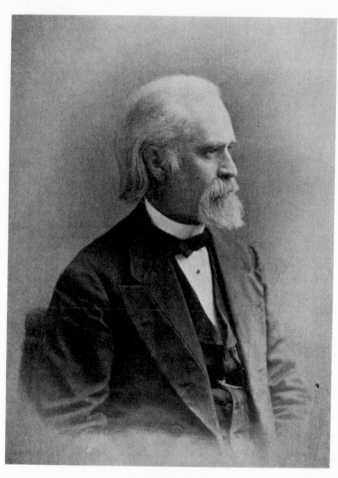

BENJAMIN DWIGHT

spent hours reading the plays, neglecting to prepare my lessons. I extracted from many of the plays quotations that impressed me, and covered the fly leaves of the volume with them, noting act and scene in which they occurred.

I cannot take leave of the High School at Clinton without further mention of Benjamin W. Dwight, its founder; he was both scholar and educator. As a pioneer in the science of language he wrote his volumes on "Modern Philology," which were among the first to draw attention to this science in our country. As an educator he was eminent both by tradition and inheritance, but even more by his own achievements; his work as director in the high schools he established at Brooklyn and at Clinton was creative, and in them he dedicated himself successfully for fifteen years to the work of inspiring young men with true ideals of life. His later years he gave to genealogy, publishing two volumes each upon the lineage of the Dwight and Strong families—those of his father and mother. Finally, his rugged candor, honesty of soul, and uprightness of character formed the crowning virtues of his life.

For three years I pursued the curriculum of the Rural High School, a course which at the time I felt was strenuous, and the benefits of which I was to realize in later life. The religious teaching I there acquired was to undergo modification. In the summer and fall of 1860, while I was at home on vacation, the presidential campaign of Lincoln, as mentioned above, was under way. Political agitation, discussion of slavery, and the threatened secession of the southern states were absorbing topics. The summer of 1861 I spent at home. Three years at the Dwight School had prepared our class for entrance to Yale, but it was decided I should not go at once; fifteen was considered too early an age, and the clouds of war were rapidly gathering. In July of that summer, when the armies were finally confronting each other in Virginia, and news of an engagement came, I remember riding in haste with my father to a nearby town to get the earliest possible information. The news, when it came, told of the humiliating defeat of the Union troops at Bull Run; in dismay and dejection we drove home, but the defeat in this first skirmish aroused still greater resolution in loyal souls. The One Hundred and Twelfth Regiment of Volunteers was raised in Chautauqua County, and one company came largely from Forestville; in visiting the camp at Jamestown, I remember how ardent was my wish that I were one of this favored group who would soon know the thrill of actual warfare.

Eighteen-sixty and sixty-one were years of stirring events in the nation. The election of Lincoln, the secession of eleven southern states, the firing on Sumter, and Lincoln's call for volunteers—these happenings and the surge of the great wave of patriotism which swept through the North reached every town and village. When the gallant young Colonel Ellsworth was shot and killed in pulling down the Confederate flag at Alexandria, Virginia, many a school boy joined in singing "We're Coming Father Abraham," and longed to be one of the seventy-five thousand volunteers to march upon the South.

In March, 1862, my father passed from earthly life. He was a man in the best sense; his inheritance and opportunities had been honorable though humble, and much had he made of them. Upright he was in character, indomitable in industry, kindly and genial in humor. His faults seem to me to have been few; he was slow in speech, moderate in ambition. He was happy in this, and in all things the better, that for twenty-six years he was blessed by a good wife, lovely in person and character, to whom he was a devoted husband. In the summer after my father's death, I cultivated the garden, of which he had been very fond; but I was too inexpert to meet with much success. That autumn I went to Silver Creek and gained a varied experience by "clerking" in a store in which my father's estate had an interest. It was a general store, with many departments; and I became familiar with its stock of drugs, groceries, confectionery, cigars, medicinal wines and liquors.

A quaint old German watch and clock maker occupied a corner in our store, a Württemberger, named Steiger. Many were the chats I had with him—broken English on his side, imperfect German on mine. Steiger told me of his native city, Ulm, upon the Danube, and further enlarged my German vocabulary. I was impressed with his story of the Ulm cathedral, stupendous in its capacity, able to accommodate thirty thousand people, and containing the greatest organ in Germany, whose sixty-four foot pipes, when fully opened and played, caused such vibration that the organist was not allowed to use them. (This must have been due to temporary construction; in 1890 the cathedral was completed.) I learned that Ulm was the home of the Meistersinger.

In 1863 our store was transferred to Forestville and combined with the village post-office. I became a servant of Uncle Sam and an amateur pharmacist, the departments other than drugs having been eliminated. My activities behind the counter had, in my own view, been intended as a bridge from school to college; books were my chief interest, and my prepossessions made of me but a mediocre salesman. I had no skill in persuading people to buy things they did not need, nor had I the enterprise of the present-day salesman, who considers one sale only a stepping-stone to the next.

We were all absorbed in the events of the Civil War (the conflict now referred to as the "War between the States"). Not being eighteen, and not having the ingenuity of the Ohio youth (afterward United States Senator Foraker) who inscribed the figure 18 on the soles of his boots and declared he was "over eighteen," it was not for me to go to war. It was my desire to go to college, and the autumn of 1863 found me again in the Rural High School at Clinton. A year of study followed. Use of tobacco, given a trial, had little appeal; I had experimented to my satisfaction with a clay pipe clandestinely in a corner of the mill at the age of eleven. Likewise the taste of beer I found repugnant. That year, too, at our school was organized one of the earliest of the high-school fraternities, the Upsilon Beta, of which I became a member. At the end of the school year in 1864, I took the college entrance examination and was admitted to Hamilton College, Clinton. That June at the College commencement I heard Elihu Root, valedictorian of the class then graduating, deliver his oration, a brilliant example of the *ore rotundo*, which did credit to Hamilton's professor of rhetoric, Anson J. Upson, under whose instruction several eloquent lawyers and preachers were developed.

I now went west, not "to grow up with the country," but because my family had moved from New York to the state of Michigan. When autumn came, I decided to enter the University of Michigan, at Ann Arbor. In September, then, of 1864, I entered the College of Arts, one of a besieging student army that numbered many hundreds. To me, looking backward as through a magic telescope, Ann Arbor appears now as a happy valley, bathed in the sunshine of golden opportunity. The classics then held the center of the stage; Henry S. Frieze and James R. Boise, pre-eminent scholars in Latin and Greek, and Andrew D. White, in history, aroused our enthusiasm. English was taught for its own sake by the famous Moses Coit Tyler, not to foster expertness in journalism or in the psychology and trickery of advertising. Alexander Winchell, famous successor to Asa Gray, held the intense interest of his classes in zoölogy and botany. He was an early advocate of the theory of evolution, then beginning to arouse the world of science and produce consternation among the orthodox. The accomplished professor occupying the chair of mathematics was Edward Olney; if he did not successfully guide me through the intricacies of algebra and the differential calculus, the fault was none of his.

There was no stadium then; the "gym" was the

CLASSMATES, ANN ARBOR, 1868

open field. Intercollegiate contests in athletics and debating were scarcely known; co-eds did not exist; Rhodes scholars had not been born. "Gosh," I can hear the modern youth exclaim, "what a dull existence." Yet, had he been there, he would have found exercise for wit and muscle; that simpler, elder day had much to recommend it.

We were always conscious of the tragic background of the Civil War. Some comrades and classmates had come from service in the field; and there were vacant chairs in the classroom, and in the ranks of the faculty as well, of those absent at the front and of some who had crossed the firing-line into eternity.

I spent two years in the literary college. Aside from absorption in the usual routine of study, there was much pleasant companionship. In the intervals of more serious work, music was for me a favorite diversion. Four young men, including myself, formed an Arion Quartette, and our songs were in request at various gatherings; we became part of the choir in a church where Professor Henry S. Frieze, a master of harmony as well as of Latin literature, played the organ. I had been pledged to the Sigma Phi fraternity at Hamilton at the end of my Clinton days; I had almost at once, on entering Ann Arbor, been offered, and had all but accepted, membership in another

Greek-letter society. Now came members of the Ann Arbor Sigma Phi, urging me to join their ranks. I found them very congenial and listened when they pressed the priority of their claim. "Ragging" of one fraternity by another was not unknown, and was winked at when it occurred. All things considered, I decided to join the Sigma Phi and take the consequences. These were never unpleasant. In the society I had chosen, I found a lifelong bond most congenial, even precious in the friendships and associations it brought.[2] In my Sophomore year, the reading of Homer and Horace opened a fascinating world of classical lore; there was high inspiration, too, in the literature of the great historians, essayists, and novelists whose works made known the treasures of minds of the past ages. I studied the great poets and, under their seductive influence, dropped into an attempt of my own at poetic expression. I find in the *University Magazine* of those years outcroppings of youthful fancy long forgotten.

"Primavera"

Through all the gnarled and oaken wold, the leaf
That shook all winter in the hurrying blast,
Though dead, upon the bough still clinging fast,
Emblem of Hope that wanton doth deceive

[2] In March, 1927, the Sigma Phi celebrated with the parent-chapter at Union College, Schenectady, New York, its one-hundredth anniversary. Elihu Root was the chief speaker on this occasion.

Yet will not utterly the heart bereave,
Falls to the teeming earth, pushed off at last
By buds that now expanding fast,
Soon round the hill a garment green will weave.
What spirit is it that doth move so bright
Through gloomy intervals of darksome wood—
Doth rehabilitate and clothe with light
Each glade, how dull so e'er its wintry mood?
We cannot know, save that we feel it flows
From that vast source whence first all life arose.

Among these was a rhyme which took a prize;
it began:

> Let every student fill his bowl
> With something not too strong, Sir.

There was also a "Parting Song for the Class of
'68," to the tune of "Maid of Athens." In 1868,
though I had left them to study medicine, I heard
my class, then graduating, sing this "Parting
Song."

The class of 1868 comprised an unusual number of men who won distinction in after life. It
must be admitted, however, that in after-years,
when its members showed a disposition to plume
themselves, men from other classes indulged in
invidious scoffing and told of meeting sixty-
eighters in the outside world who were anything
but a credit to the boasters. Of the forty-two
members graduated, there were twelve who
achieved high honors—scholastic, scientific, edu-

cational. Nine occupied chairs as heads of departments in the Universities of Michigan, Wisconsin, and Chicago, in the departments of Latin, Greek, English, history, and zoölogy. Three were important architects and engineers. Other members were eminent in law, medicine, and judicial positions; also as educators and on boards of public administration. Mark Harrington, though later he suffered a mental eclipse, was professor of astronomy and director of the Observatory at Ann Arbor, afterward weather chief at Washington, D.C., and president of the State University of Washington. Boardman, publisher of the weekly *Railroad Gazette*, had his office in Chicago, but in 1871, after the great fire, transferred his business to New York; there was no break in the coming-out of the weekly issues. The *Gazette* was, for more than twenty years, an important railway authority of the country. Demmon, successor to Moses Coit Tyler in the department of English at the University of Michigan, was an authority on libraries. Several members of the class served with distinction in the Civil War. Two were United States consuls in Europe; one was engineer of sanitation in the Columbian Exposition. Walter, who perished in the sinking of the "Bourgogne," July, 1898, was known for his scholarship in Latin and the Romance languages.

I have mentioned the change in direction of my

studies which I made at the end of my second year. The means at my command—rather, the lack of means—made early preparation for active life advisable. After long meditation I had chosen medicine as the profession most consonant with my aptitudes, and in the autumn of 1866 transferred to the Medical College of the University of Michigan. At this time I wrote a playlet, entitled "Mary, the Male-clad Medical Student." It was prompted by the discussion, frequent then, as to the fitness of woman for the study and practice of medicine. In that dark day, admission of women to this profession was practically unheard of. The prologue of my playlet began with these lines:

> How long must injured woman wait
> In sackcloth before Science's gate?

As a student I had taken part in the discussion of the subject by sending to the New York *Nation* an article in which I advocated certain specialties as especially appropriate for women physicians (internal medicine, obstetrics, gynecology), asserting that woman's competence in these would be equal to that of men, and stating my belief that in major surgery she would be at a disadvantage. As the matter stood at that time, this was the advanced position. The courses in the University of Michigan Medical School consisted chiefly of theoretical instruction; this was true of other schools of medicine in that day. In the chemical laboratory and the dissecting room, it is true, theory was put into practice; but books and lectures absorbed most of the student's attention. Each student was expected to have a preceptor, a practitioner, with whom the time intervening between courses was spent in gaining knowledge of the practical side of the profession. Ann Arbor, then a town of a few thousand inhabitants, did not possess hospitals and clinical facilities equal to those of the larger cities. Our school, however, gave opportunities which in that day were unsurpassed anywhere in the country for what are now called the premedical branches of study.

The foundation stones of medicine, anatomy, and physiology were for me well laid and thoroughly established by a teacher who could with difficulty be equaled in his time or in any time, Corydon L. Ford, supreme master of his subject, who possessed a genius for clear demonstration and for enlisting and holding the interest of his hearers. For forty years his teaching on the intricate functions of the organs of the human body threw clear light upon the path of the students before him, in their preparation for entering the field of medicine. The beginner has always had a tremendous task in memorizing

Gray's *Anatomy of the Human Body;* in learning the names of thousands of bones, muscles, nerves, lymphatics; of organs, glands, secretions. I questioned whether Gray possessed a single sympathetic nerve, and addressed an ode to Henry Gray, F.R.S., author of "Gray's Anatomy, an Ode," in which I pronounced maledictions upon him for the torture to which, through him, untold generations of hapless medicos were doomed.

There were other inspiring teachers: Professor Moses Gunn held the chair of surgery; aside from his brilliant attainments as a surgeon and lecturer, his animation and humor often enlivened his lectures; he invited questions and often answered with interjections of spicy comment. He was later called to the chair of surgery in Rush Medical College, now School of Medicine of the University of Chicago. Professor Alonzo Palmer discoursed ably on internal medicine. Dr. Abram Sager, professor of gynecology, had rare ability in clear demonstration. The course in chemistry, organic and inorganic, given under Professor Albert Prescott was advanced for the time. Bacteriology and antisepsis had not then been born; microscopy was in its infancy; Virchow's cellular pathology was beginning to work as a leaven; but twenty years were to pass before the hygienic laboratory was established under Victor Vaughn.

The doctrine of evolution was then just beginning to disturb the equanimity of the theological world. The assault upon the Book of Genesis was met with alarm and opposition in some quarters; was accepted in others. The assumption that man had developed from the brute creation, more especially from simian ancestry, occasioned violent controversy and dealt a violent blow to the belief that *Homo sapiens* was a special creation, formed in the image of God, and had dwelt on earth less than ten thousand years. That evolution had been at work for aeons, for hundreds of thousands of years, was inconceivable to the thought of that day. Herbert Spencer's agnosticism was felt to be synonymous with atheism.

My people were now interested in a tract of pine wood in western Michigan. There logs were being cut and floated down the Black River to the sawmill at South Haven, to be turned into lumber for the Chicago market. The sawmill afforded me an opportunity for employment in the vacation seasons; and for two summers during my course in medicine I helped myself along by working there, learned how the buzz saw worked, and became familiar with this new kind of mill. My nights and free days were given to study and reading. I enjoyed occasional outings on lake and river in that pleasant country, largely virgin forest. Even then orchards were beginning to be developed, for it had been found that the peach could be grown here in perfection, owing to the mildness of the winter climate and the warm current of the lake. The green, unripe peaches were sent in schooner loads across the lake to the city market; but one who had known only the sharp taste of the "hard" fruit could not imagine the delicious flavor of the fully ripened Michigan peach. One summer I enjoyed a trip to Chicago on the schooner; by a lucky chance there was an opera troupe in town, and with immense enjoyment I heard *The Barber of Seville.*

I obtained my medical degree in the spring of 1869. Hospital experience was the next requirement. A proposal from a colleague, then finishing a year of service at the Brooklyn (New York) City Hospital, attracted me, and I resolved to enter the competitive examination to be held in July for one of the four internships. I read and studied without intermission from March to mid-July, taking the standard textbooks in each department of medicine and measuring out the number of pages for each day to take me through the work. I passed the examination successfully and entered upon my duty as intern August first. Six months were to be spent in the medical wards, and six in the surgical. I obtained here valuable practical experience in the medicine and surgery of the day. The revolution wrought by germ discoveries and antisepsis was just in its beginning. The microscope, clinical thermometer, ophthalmoscope, and other instruments of precision which were soon to be accepted as a matter of course were becoming known but were not generally employed; we were dependent more upon keen observation and close study of physical signs than upon artificial aids. Service in the Brooklyn Hospital afforded valuable experience in the field of internal medicine, which was then not organized in a diversity of specialties; in surgery, the emergency and maternity wards offered opportunity, as did the special wards for colored patients and for sailors, maintained under government contract. In these last named, venereal disease was the predominating ailment. In the midst of my absorbing work in the Hospital, I remember an event of that autumn which made a deep impression: "Black Friday," September 24. It grew out of the disastrous "cornering" of the gold market in New York by a conspiracy in which Jay Gould and "Jim" Fiske were implicated. Panic and widespread ruin resulted, also huge dishonest fortunes for the conspirators.

The proximity of New York gave access to clinics and lectures by the masters in many fields. I would here name some of the eminent men in the medical world of that period. Austin Flint and Alonzo Clark in the Bellevue and Physicians and Surgeons' schools, respectively, were leading masters in the practice of medicine. Willard Parker was an authority in the genito-urinary diseases; he was a humanitarian also, and was made successor to Valentine Mott, director of the first state inebriate asylum, at Binghamton, New York. He maintained there was no food or medicinal value in alcohol, a novel doctrine in his day. Another famous surgeon was James R. Wood, who, with Willard Parker, had a strong hand in converting the old disreputable Bellevue Alms House into a hospital of the first rank, and later in establishing the Bellevue Hospital Medical College, in which Wood was a most popular and successful teacher. The Wood Museum, created by him, was a collection of rare and instructive anatomical and pathological specimens. Marion Sims was pre-eminent for his genius in inventing instruments and in applying their use in operations designed to cure the diseases of women; among them was one that had been regarded as well-nigh incurable: vesicovaginal fistula. His success in this operation had been such that not only in this country but in France and England he was invited to operate; honors were conferred upon him by learned societies. During the Franco-Prussian War, while I was serving in the German field hospital at Pont à Mousson, he was organizing in France the Anglo-American Ambulance Corps.

Still another New York specialist acknowledged as a master in his field was Frank Hamilton, to whom fractures and dislocations were as an open book. Many new methods and appliances were devised by him, and his book on the subject was an authority. He was the consultant called to attend President Garfield after his assassination, but found the President's spinal column wounded beyond his or any power to cure. Lewis A. Sayre, of the same faculty as Hamilton, was a great orthopedist; was the first to use plaster-of-Paris jackets in spinal diseases and curvature and, I think, to practice suspension by the neck in spinal scoliosis. His profanity in the presence of nurses would perhaps scarcely be noticed in the present day.

I would mention also some of the men of note in that day whose practice was in the department of nervous and mental disease, to which my own labors were afterward directed: William A. Hammond, found to have been unjustly dismissed from his position as surgeon-general during the Civil war, was reinstated by Congress in 1879. During his surgeon-generalship, he established the army medical museum and was professor of diseases of the mind and nervous system in Bellevue Hospital Medical College. He wrote with authority on psychopathology. Dr. John P. Gray was at this time also lecturing at Bellevue Hospital Medical College; he was a pioneer in psychiatry, head of the Utica New York State Hospital for the Insane. He had been the main reliance as expert in the prosecution of Guiteau for the murder of President Garfield, pronouncing Guiteau "sane and responsible," in opposition to the opinion of E. C. Spitzka, who pronounced him "insane." Dr. S. Weir Mitchell, of Philadelphia, occupied a pre-eminent position both at home and abroad as a neurologist. The foundation of his fame in this specialty was laid during the Civil War, when he took charge of Turner's Lane, a hospital for patients afflicted with injuries of nerves and brain. There he gained illuminating experiences and made deep study of the functions of the nervous system. He possessed a genius for research and for the formulation of successful treatment of nervous maladies; as an example of this we have the method of treatment for nervous exhaustion and hysteria which came to be known as the "Weir Mitchell Rest Cure." Patients often responded to this cure with what seemed magical alacrity. It was in reality an application of psychotherapy, though in that day the term was not used. Dr. Mitchell was known also for his secular writings, especially as the author of the novel *Hugh Wynne*.

Apart from professional interests, I recall other

events of the winter of 1869–70: There was in
New York a Shakespearean revival, the production of *Hamlet* by two well-known actors of the
day—by Edwin Booth at his own theater, and by
the English actor Fechter at the Winter Garden.
Fechter was rotund, blue-eyed, and played the
part in a blond curly wig; this was in sharp contrast to Edwin Booth's more solemn, classical
portrayal. At the same time, the comedian Fox
was presenting at a third theater a burlesque of
Hamlet, amusing to "groundlings" but painful to
the discerning. At Central Park Garden, Theo-
dore Thomas' orchestra concerts were attracting
enthusiastic audiences. His assemblage of players was the origin of the orchestra destined to
develop into the now famous Symphony Orchestra of Chicago.

It happened that on August 1, 1870, the day
upon which my year of service at the Brooklyn
City Hospital ended, an opportunity came to me
to engage as volunteer assistant surgeon in the
military service of Germany. On July 19 the
Franco-Prussian War had begun; the rapid succession of battles in the first weeks of the war had
proved sanguinary to such a degree that the surgical resources of Germany had been found
wholly inadequate to provide care for the
wounded. In this emergency the German consul
in New York had been authorized by his govern-

ment to engage American surgeons who could speak German. On the morning of August first, I saw in the paper a notice of this fact and lost no time in making application. My application was accepted; this narrative will therefore continue with an account of my experience in field and reserve hospitals in France and Germany.

CHAPTER TWO

*Experiences of an American Volunteer
Assistant Surgeon in the Franco-
Prussian War, 1870-71*

AN ACCOUNT is here presented of the experiences of a young American practitioner of medicine who was engaged as volunteer surgeon in the Franco-Prussian War of 1870 and 1871.

At the time of my arrival in France in the second week of September, 1870, the decisive battles of the war had been fought and won by the German armies. Napoleon III, with Marshall MacMahon and his entire army of more than eighty thousand, had been made prisoner at Sedan. Marshall Bazaine, defeated at Gravelotte, had been forced, with his army of one hundred and seventy thousand, to take refuge in Metz. What remained of military operations consisted of certain minor engagements and the advance upon Paris for the siege, which lasted through the winter of 1870 and 1871. There was no opportunity for one who arrived after September first to participate in field-of-battle activities, but there was abundant opportunity for service in attending the wounded in the field and reserve hospitals of Germany: in Hessen Cassel, where I was assigned, and later in Wilhelmshoehe, the place of Napoleon's imprisonment. In April, service ended with honorable discharge and award of a medal *Für Pflichttreue im Kriege*. My way then lay, both by inclination and duty, to Berlin, where world-interests centered; there also my account with the government was to be settled. Arrival there was followed by a stay during the spring and summer, which gave opportunity for rare experiences: seeing the peace treaty presented by Bismarck and hearing it discussed in the Reichstag; meeting the American ambassador and famous historian, George Bancroft; encountering frequently upon the streets the talked-of personages of the day, Czar Alexander and Kaiser Wilhelm I, as they rode in Unter den Linden; seeing great bodies of troops reviewed; hearing the opera which Berlin offered in those days of her triumph; and finally matriculating at the University of Berlin for Virchow's course in microscopy.

On June 16, 1871, took place the triumphal return of the army to Berlin and the celebration of the victory of the recovery of Alsace and Lorraine, the establishment of the German Empire. Forty thousand troops with the Kaiser, Field

Marshall von Moltke, and General von Roon at their head, marched the length of Unter den Linden; royal and imperial personages followed, then infantry, cavalry, and artillery in gala uniform; the ladies of the court in open carriages.

To return to the August days of 1870: when the consul had referred me for medical and linguistic qualifications to a well-known German-American practitioner uptown in New York, who, after an interview, gave his recommendation, I was notified to appear on August 13 and to complete arrangements for sailing that day from New York on the steamship "Columbia" of the Anchor Line. With four other doctors engaged by the consul as I had been, and several Germans returning under military orders to the Fatherland, I boarded the "Columbia," bearing papers of "legitimation" signed by Otto von Bismarck, chancellor of the Nord Deutscher Bund. Two weeks' sailing found us in Glasgow, where we spent Sunday; saw the shipyards of Greenock; partook of salmon from the Clyde; and found Sabbath observance so strict that our indulgence in the singing of secular songs was taboo in our hotel, although there were many men on the streets who showed the effects of their Saturday-night debauch. We crossed to Edinburgh; sailed thence from Leith Harbor for Rotterdam. There

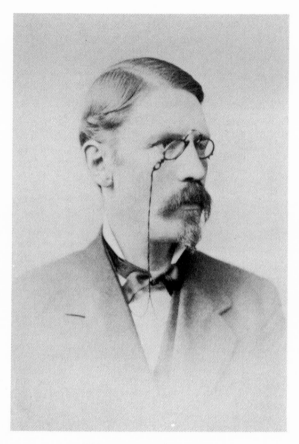

RICHARD DEWEY, 1871

we were referred to the Herr Oberst of the nearby fortress of Wesel, who ordered us to the headquarters of the Seventh Army Corps at Münster, capital of Westphalia.

Arriving after business hours in Münster, we put up for the night at a *Gasthof*. The first event next day was breakfast; and as we had heard of the excellence of Westphalian ham (*Schinken*), we ordered ham and eggs for breakfast. In due course, cold sliced ham was brought with poached eggs—*Spiegeleir*, or "glazed eggs," the Germans call them. Our German was put to a test in explaining, but finally we got fried ham and eggs. The lieutenant colonel at army headquarters issued the wished-for transportation orders to take us to the front; they were addressed to the Seventh Army Corps in the field at Pont-à-Mousson in Lorraine; at last we could anticipate active service. The journey took us through Cologne, where we arrived on Saturday night, September third. We found the waiting-rooms of the station filled with cots occupied by wounded. Tense excitement filled the air caused by the news recently received of the capture that day of Napoleon at Sedan. Emerging from the station, we came directly into the public square in front of the great cathedral, where, in celebration, an immense bonfire had been lighted. Every window in the square was illuminated; bands were playing; flags waving; people marching and singing "Heil dir im Siegeskranz." A shrill cornet was playing "Red dawn that lights me to my grave." Strains of "Wacht am Rhein," "Deutschland über Alles," and of folk songs sung by excited marching groups filled the air. The silent grandeur of the great cathedral contrasted strangely with the tumult; the sublime twin towers rising hundreds of feet seemed to have upon them the red glow of war; the strident jubilation was like an echo from the fields of battle. The event did indeed signify the defeat of the French. The surrender, in figures, meant 82,000 men killed, wounded, missing, or taken prisoner; 558 pieces of ordnance captured; and enough of the French chassepot rifles to replace the inferior German needle-gun for the army in the field. The vociferous rejoicings were protracted far into the night, and there was little sleep in the hotel where we were quartered; but morning found us at the Rhine Railroad station ready to board train for the front in France.

As our train went forward along the border of the Rhine, we saw vine-clad hills glowing in the autumn sun with the majestic river at their base; the Siebengebirge and the lofty peak of the Drachenfels came into view, calling to mind the legend of Siegfried and the cave of the fiery dragon. But from thought of legend and romance we

were rudely recalled to reality and the grim circumstance of war. Our train was now shunted to
a siding to let a long procession of cars pass forward, rushing to the front with supplies. In a
short time we were again upon the switch, this
time for a train moving in the opposite direction
—a long line of coaches loaded with prisoners of
war bound for confinement in the fortresses of the
interior; we caught glimpses of crestfallen figures
at doors and windows. On the floors of open flat
cars crouched swarthy Algerian "Turcos," guarded by armed Prussian soldiers. It was a journey
of frequent interruptions, in which we were constantly stirred by spectacles of war on one hand
and by the marvels of the German scene on the
other. At Coblenz, we saw the great fortress
Ehrenbreitstein, crowning the heights across the
Rhine; here the billion of indemnity exacted
from France at the end of the war was later to be
safeguarded. Near St. Goar we recalled the story
of the cruel Lorelei.

Our first real stopping-place was Saarbrücken.
On alighting we were struck by the battered appearance of the station—holes in the brick walls,
the glass roof over the platform shattered. This
had been the scene of the first engagement of the
war, on August second; here the young crown
prince had received, as his father boasted, his
"baptism of fire," and Louis Napoleon had sent

a magniloquent dispatch recounting it to the
Empress Eugénie. The engagement, really only a
skirmish, had been almost the only engagement
in which success attended the French arms. Here
in the station were hospital beds occupied by
wounded; in the station yard a stricken family,
driven from their home.

At St. Johan across the Saar, the commandant
had in us a problem; no other Americans with papers like ours had come his way. He informed us
suavely that he must consult headquarters. We
waited three days in this quiet town. On the
third, instructions came: we were to be sent to
Remilly, where transportation to Pont à Mousson on the Moselle, headquarters of our Army
Medical Corps, would be provided. This journey, though it was but thirty miles, required the
most of two days; one slept in the baggage net-
ting with a coat for pillow. We passed the battle
fields of Forbach and St. Avold, where the people
were again at their usual labors, the peasant
women doing their washing in the streams and
carrying the laden tubs balanced on their heads.
Women were working in the fields, a novel sight
to American eyes. On September 8, in rain, we
reached Pont à Mousson, having been supplied
with *Ordonnanz* (*schwarzbrod*, bacon, and salt),
and having been given the rank of officers of the

medical corps. Our covered wagon gave shelter but allowed little view of the country.

My narrative may here be continued by the inclusion of a letter written by me on October 17, 1870, and published in the New York *Nation*:[1]

"Some observations made in connection with the two military hospitals where I have been serving, one in France and one in Germany, may give your readers some idea of these institutions as brought into existence by the war now in progress. A brief account is sent herewith of some experiences in L'Hopital de la Seminaire, at Pont à Mousson on the Moselle in Lorraine, and in the Royal Reserve Hospital, No. 11, at Cassel.

"Early in September, riding into Pont à Mousson one dark rainy evening, I noticed, crossing the stone bridge which here spans the Moselle, a large church from whose spacious windows lights were shining. It was late for evening service, yet, thought I, perhaps the afflicted people are prolonging their supplications or rehearsing some Miserere with a new sense of its meaning. Soon I learned the truth, for I joined until beyond midnight in the services held there. The assemblage was composed of about five hundred wounded

[1] Permission has been given by the editors of the *Nation* to use here such letters as were published by them.

soldiers, French and Prussian; the services were directed by half a dozen surgeons, and a force of Sisters of Charity. The sermon was uttered by tongues speaking from the mangled flesh of injured men. The church is a fine large structure in the renaissance style, built side by side with a seminary of similar style and dimensions, the two being connected by spacious wings; colonnades traverse their length, enclosing a handsome inner court. The whole, known as the Seminaire, was formerly a flourishing Catholic Divinity School. It is now converted into two immense field hospitals, accommodating nearly one thousand patients. When the Prussians took possession of the town, they found the spot deserted, offering accommodations of every sort requisite: large airy dormitories; apartments for surgeons, officers and nurses; housekeeping equipment; even an elaborate garden, whose arbor it was necessary to convert into a morgue. Many of the windows command a fine view of the Moselle. In the court, pavilions have been erected for the accommodation of contagious and infectious diseases. Only a few hundred mattresses were required to make the hospital ready for its inmates; and inmates came in overwhelming numbers. Pont à Mousson is the center to which wounded are brought from all the battle fields to the southwest of Metz; wagon trains are constantly arriving, and fill to capacity the eight field hospitals the town provides. At the Seminaire, the wounded are first received in the church itself, and are laid upon the straw-covered floor. When they arrive in trains of hundreds at a time, it requires the whole night to attend to their needs; one can scarcely find a path among them as they lie; halls, porticoes and wings are packed to their utmost. From the church the wounded are distributed as their cases require: the transportable are sent back to the reserve hospitals of Germany; the more severe cases retained in the Seminaire; those having internal injuries are assigned to the appropriate localities; those with contagious disease to the Pavilions. When the beds become scarce, it is the French who are laid on straw on the floors of the halls.

"The wounds of the Prussian soldiers, inflicted by the Chassepot rifle, are remarkable for the straight and uncompromising lines which they present. At point-blank range, the missile of this weapon makes a staight line through whatever objects come in its way, not deviating as do balls of inferior rifles. Thus are seen wounds through the width of the hand, the ball having shattered every one of the five bones in its course; wounds through both thighs, fracturing one of them; wounds through all the bones of the pelvis, or through those of the face and skull, made with undeviating directness. The Prussians acknowledge the superiority of the Chassepot arm, and have equipped regiments of their own with those taken from prisoners.

"In the Seminaire, the duties of the nurse are performed exclusively by the various orders, Catholic and Protestant, of the Sisters of Mercy and Charity. In the Church and lower rooms, Sisters of the Society of Jesus from the Rhine provinces, and Sisters of the Order of Saint Francis from Westphalia are employed. All of the Jesuit Sisters speak French, and are hence best employed in the care of the French. In the upper rooms the intelligent and faithful Protestant deaconesses from Berlin and from Rhenish Prussia are in charge, under Professor Roser, a surgeon of wide reputation from the University of Marburg. The chief business of the Dispensaries has been to provide sanitation, leaving the restoration of health, after the surgeon has done all he can, to the healing power of nature: good food, good air and nursing are relied upon. The number of capital operations made at this hospital at first was very large: amputations, resections of skull fractures, ligations of major blood vessels, were the order of the day. Operations are performed under carbolic spray. The unfortunate subjects of these operations have not done as well as we could wish, and for reasons which are not far to seek. They arrive here after the most favorable time has passed, having lain sometimes for days, near the fields where they fell, or in farm houses or sheds wherever room could be made for them. Hence although they have here the benefit of whatever skill and care can do, progress is unfavorable, and numbers are carried off by one or another of the pests which prey upon humanity in wartime. When recently in the Seminaire it was desired to separate the French from the German wounded, and the question was put to them as to their nationality, some of the French replied: 'moitié Français; moitié Allemand.' It appeared on inquiry that these were thoughtless boys or Algerians, who thought that by pretending to be German they would get better treatment."

Another *Nation* letter follows, which deals with the surgical service in the German Army hospitals:

"Until the outbreak of this war, the Prussian Army has had for a battalion of infantry (one thousand men), two surgeons; there were thus six surgeons to one of its colossal regiments of three thousand men, or one to each five hundred. In the cavalry and artillery the proportion is somewhat greater: one surgeon to two hundred men. This provision has been wholly inadequate to the present emergency, and there are at present more than two hundred extra surgeons as well as a considerable number of volunteers and assistants of various degrees. Private Prussian practitioners of skill and repute have been induced by the Government's solicitation as well as by their own humanity to join the army, and high special commissions have been created for them. I met in the Hospital at Pont à Mousson German, English, American, Austrian, Swiss, and Russian surgeons and doctors. The Swiss Government sent thirty surgeons to the field, fifteen to the French and fifteen to the German side. An army corps of forty thousand men now has sixty surgeons and provision for twelve field hospitals, each accommodating two hundred men, and supplied with five surgeons, thirty krankentrager (stretcher bearers), and a proportionate number of nurses, assistants, ambulances and carriers of supplies. One half of the force is stationed directly at the rear of the army and does for the wounded whatever the immediate emergency may require. The other half is established with the second station, where major operations are performed. Here blood flows freely and the red blouse with which the surgeon envelopes his uniform is sadly typical in its hue. In this second station the wounded are retained until their removal is dictated by prudence or demanded by necessity—more often the

latter; for after many of the recent battles it has
been impossible to find shelter or beds for the in-
coming wounded until some of the emergency
hospitals in churches, barns, farm houses or inns,
had been evacuated. The cold and rainy weather
of which we had so much, made such journeys
doubly painful and disastrous, and the number
who have breathed their last upon the straw,
jolting across the country in the wagons, if it
could be known would be a tragic commentary on
the Prussian Army's provision for its wounded.
Nothing however is to be said in disparagement
of the merits of the army surgeons; their zeal and
ability are too well known to need confirmation;
and it may be said that foresight could not have
anticipated or prevented this misery and loss.
Moreover, as we cannot hope that the days of the
world's wars are over, we have the satisfaction of
knowing that a lesson has been learned, whose
value in military surgery the future will show.

"In speaking of the German army surgeons,
one gladly pays tribute of respect to their science
and skill, as well as to their courage and esprit de
corps. Such men as Lagenbeck, Strohmeyer and
Roser represent these qualities with distinction.
As a body they have almost universally discarded
the red cross of the International Convention,
scorning to be considered non-combatants. One
of the assistant surgeons, as he was attending the

wounded on the battle field of Wörth, was shot by a stray ball through his eye; he coolly took out his handkerchief, and binding the wound proceeded with his work. When he had completed in an orderly manner his care of the wounded man, he gave him into the charge of the *krankentrager* and returned to the hospital; there it was found that his eye had been completely destroyed. As a reward for his intrepidity, he was presented with the decoration of the "Iron Cross" by the hand of the King. I may be allowed a few words on German operative surgery and surgical appliances, as compared with those of our own country. The Germans are pre-eminent in deep investigation and thorough information; but in candor, one may say an American is not led to think less highly of the surgeons and surgery of his own country. One who has seen and studied practical surgery in any of the chief American Hospitals will scarcely see here order, skillful manipulation, rapidity and brilliancy in as great a degree as he is accustomed to see them at home. In the operating room there is more or less confusion; the preliminaries do not seem to have been fully planned; all of the required instruments are not at hand for the operator; and no one person is charged with the duty of handling them. When the surgeon calls for an instrument often more than one will attempt to comply with the request.

Those who look on discuss the various steps freely and not in quiet tones, offering any suggestions
that occur to them. Their instruments, though in
general made of finer steel than we get in America, seem clumsy in appearance and construction
and are not so well adapted to the hand. The
American models of the more common instruments exceed the German in elegance.

There is moreover a lack of many convenient
ingenious contrivances which are to be found in
American Hospitals, and it is amusing to see the
air of lofty indifference with which the German
officer listens to any suggestion of the possibility
of methods or apparatus which excel his own; for
there is in the average German a quite percepti-
ble condescension when other countries as compared with Germany are in discussion. A com-
parison of the hospital wards of the two countries
in the matter of convenience, neatness and order
would it seems to me result favorably for America; indeed they appear to concern themselves little here about externals; yet even if one's impression is less favorable, if he looks closely he finds
that the essentials have been well attended to;
that results are creditable. Some allowance should
perhaps be made for the exigencies of war; but
the surgeons here considered are those of the first
rank. The Hospitals too in the large towns of
France, like Pont à Mousson and Nancy, are now

fully equipped, for every facility is at hand for such equipment, according to German standards. The depot of supplies, under the direction of the *Johanniter Ritter* Society, has at Saarbrücken been enabled by the liberal contributions from every part of Europe, as well as from America, to meet every demand for materials required. The Sisters of Mercy attend faithfully to the care of the patients. The number of doctors, surgeons and assistants who have volunteered their services is even superfluous. The wounded are now being comfortably removed in large numbers to the reserve hospitals that have been established in several of the large cities of Germany, and we begin to rejoice in the hope that the scenes of blood and suffering are over, although the reflection forces itself upon us that the most frightful suffering of war is that of the survivors—upon those maimed for life, and upon those who continue to live after all that life once offered is forever lost. Those who perished no longer suffer."

A letter telling of Christmas in wartime, written from Cassel, on December 26, 1870, follows:

"On Christmas night a train carrying eight hundred sick and wounded French prisoners arrived in Cassel, and halted that the men might have an opportunity to recover in some measure from the effects of the cold, hunger and thirst, from which in addition to their wounds, they were suffering; might have the dressings, medicines or treatment of which they stood in need. They were on their way to Berlin, whence they were to be sent still farther north, and all must be done which could help them endure the hardships still in store; for their journey in the miserable freight cars, neither lighted nor warmed, and supplied with only a scanty allowance of straw must continue through the night. Numbers had frostbitten hands, feet and faces; four were found actually, perhaps mercifully, frozen to death. The train had left Nancy two days before, when the weather, though raw, was not severe in temperature. But during the first night the cold became intense, reaching 14 to 16 degrees (Reaumur). Some of the prisoners were transported in open platform cars, with no shelter except what their miserable clothing afforded. The train had continued its route with true military observance of orders, regardless of consequences. The effect of forty-eight hours of uninterrupted suffering from cold cannot be exaggerated by the liveliest imagination; many were in such condition that it would have been fatal to send them farther. Hence a considerable number were detained at Cassel, and divided among the military hospitals of the city.

"Sixteen were assigned to the hospital where I

was engaged, and since I was on duty as 'officer of the day,' I examined them on their arrival. They required to be looked after with special reference to small-pox, for that disease had attacked some of their comrades on the way from France. There were none who showed symptoms of that fatal sickness, but all were afflicted in varying degrees with one or another of the unavoidable ills that had lain in wait for them; forty-eight hours of chill was showing its disastrous effects. Here I found the dusky countenance and partial as-phyxia of a commencing severe pneumonia; there the swollen joints and intense agony of rheumatic fever; some were exhausted victims of dysentery. Their bodies were emaciated in nearly every case, covered with eruptions, infested with ver-min. The warm bath, into which they were of necessity forced, and the fresh clothing required before they could be allowed to take their beds seemed to them cruel, a final torture to test their endurance.

"The prisoners were all from the Loire army, and had been captured in or about Orléans. Four were African 'Turcos,' wearing the picturesque Zouave uniform, stupid but good natured fellows —certainly not savage and blood-thirsty animals, as generally represented in the German press. The rest were from infantry regiments. One flaxen-haired blue-eyed 'Elsässer,' spoke German

with entire fluency, and offered in his Teuton-
ic traits, a marked contrast to the Latin pro-
clivities of his comrades. He had received a
severe gun-shot wound through the shoulder at
Moulin d'Anvilliers, before Orléans, on the third
of December, where the French made such obsti-
nate resistance, but were finally overpowered by
the Holsteiners. He seemed to win the hearts of
the German attendants, not only by his tempera-
ment and appearance which allied him so closely to them, but still more by his grit under severe
suffering, and his forlorn appearance. He acted
as interpreter to his comrades, and indeed spoke
better German than French. He was com-
plimented on his German looks and speech; as-
sured that he could now forget French entirely,
and make German his mother-tongue. He made
no reply; he had not yet learned to transfer his
allegiance to the conquerors of his country.

"A soldiers' funeral is no uncommon sight in
these times. Almost every day two or three of
them pass in the street before my window; but
this afternoon two passed whose unusual nature
perhaps merits a few words. In only one particular they were different from the procession which
ordinarily escorts the Prussian soldier to his
grave: a squad of perhaps fifty men marching in
rear and van divisions, between which are borne
upon the shoulders of six comrades the soldiers'

mortal remains. On the black-draped coffin rest the sabre and helmet of the deceased. These two processions differed from the others in that instead of the burnished Prussian helmet, encircled with wreath of immortelles, there rested upon one coffin the elaborately braided red cap of a French soldier of the line, and upon the other the tasseled head-piece of an Algerian Zouave. The bright red of these head-coverings made a striking contrast to the solemn black pall. These were two of those who recently made so disastrous a journey here from France, and it cannot be long before they will be followed by others of their comrades, many of whom are in a condition which forbids the hope of recovery.

"It will perhaps seem like cruelty or criminal neglect on the part of the government that men should be frozen to death during transportation through the country, but the circumstance was one which could not have been foreseen, and had it been, would have been difficult to prevent; the soldiers of the Prussian army are transported in precisely the same manner. The cold came on suddenly; other cars were not to be had; military orders are necessarily peremptory, and the fate which overtook these men was one of the inevitable consequences of war. At 'The Spotted Buck,' a quaint old inn near the hospital, I heard a group of soldiers and burghers talking of this. One veteran of seventy-seven years, who had been at Leipsic in 1813, as he handed his snuff-box around the table, recounted the horrors which in 'anno dreizehn' stared every wounded soldier in the face. By contrast, the loss of a few men by freezing to death seemed to him but a trifle. Altogether, the Hessians and Prussians do not find it difficult to justify the misfortunes of France; the way in which Napoleon I made these provinces a hunting-ground early in the century is not forgotten: his setting up his brother Jerome as 'King of Westphalia' in this very town of Hessen Cassel; neither are the designs forgotten which his nephew a few months ago entertained of marching upon Berlin with a victorious army.[2] On Wednesday evening of each week, the survivor of Leipsic is joined at The Spotted Buck by a comrade who fought at Waterloo. The two old companions in arms are men of place and influence in the town, and the turn their conversation takes may be imagined. Northern Hesse, under Prussia only since '66, might be restless under the Prussian military system in other circumstances, but has shown no reluctance to send men against France during the war, and has done valiant service on more than one occasion.

[2] Early in the war it was known that the French invaders, counting on victory, had drawn up a plan for the partition of Prussia and a redividing of Germany by which the Saar district was to fall to France.

The young men who are now being called into service for the first time respond as a rule with alacrity; those who are sufficiently well-to-do to meet their own expenses and are ambitious to become officers, are allowed to enter service as 'one year volunteers,' i.e. they serve a year for nothing. At its very worst, indeed, the severe but impartial and selfishly enlightened policy of the Prussian government could not but be preferable to the petty tyranny which the Hessians formerly suffered under the despotic rule of the deposed Kurfürst, Elector of Hesse. Whenever an American finds himself in the company of Prussians, he is sure to encounter, in one form or another, the question of American attitude toward the French Republic. The veteran of Leipsic in speaking on this matter permitted himself to refer to that republic by the untranslatable term, 'schweinerei,' and gave it as his firm conviction that Americans are reasonable beings, and would understand the difference between a 'schweinerei' and a genuine republic. The Germans here are generous in their recognition of the relief and rescue work administered in Paris by the American ambassador, Mr. Washburn, in the frightful circumstances incident to the siege of the city."

A letter dated May 18, 1871, from Berlin, and published in the New York *Nation*, follows:

"A half year spent in the Prussian military hospital service has called forth some reflections which may interest your readers. In Hessen Cassel, where the writer was stationed during the last few months of the war, the buildings comprising the *Train Remise* (train depot), of the 11th army corps were converted into an immense Reserve Hospital, with a capacity of nearly eight hundred beds, which were increased to one thousand by eight American Barracks—Amerikanische Barracken—erected on adjacent ground. Doktor Strohmeyer, the renowned Göttingen Professor, author of a book entitled 'Experience With Gun Shot Wounds in the Year '66,' says of the Amerikanische Barracken: "We have the Americans to thank for a current of fresh air admitted into military hospitals of modern times. . . . .' 'Hospitals were never so little crowded, and so completely furnished. . . . . They (the Americans) may be proud of their ability in having made this assertion possible.'

I had charge of one division in the Reserve Hospital (eighty beds); during the time of my engagement more than seven hundred patients passed through the division assigned to me. I had therefore a fair opportunity of seeing something of the Prussian soldier in all branches of the service and from every province of the Kingdom, as well as troops from other portions of the North German Confederation.

"One of the first things that must strike anyone who comes in contact with the Prussian private is that while he possesses in an eminent degree the virtues of the soldier, as his achievements have abundantly shown, he is free from the vices which the life of a soldier is supposed to foster, and which have generally characterized the soldier's calling. Far from being improvident, idle, blasphemous, intemperate, or lawless, he is law-abiding, highly disciplined, loyal, respectful to superiors. The impression which one gets is of simpleminded, frugal and honest men. They would be the last to disregard an order. Let me illustrate: The use of alcohol in all American and English hospitals is hedged about with strictest precautions, and in spite of these is yet constantly abused. In the hospitals of Germany on the other hand, during the war, beer or wine was supplied by the government to every patient as a part of his daily diet; and the Soldiers' Aid Society considered it an important task to provide extra quantities of these articles for such patients as were thought to need them; not wine and beer alone, but rum, brandy and whisky were easily within the reach of every patient. Yet in nearly six months among seven hundred men, although my knowledge of and daily contact with them was such that an excess of the sort would hardly have escaped notice, I met with only four cases of drunkenness (one scarcely deserving the name), and I cannot remember to have met a man who could be called a confirmed sot. On the King's birthday, the Sisters of Charity prepared liberal quantities of punch for the patients under their charge, and I am sure that a thoughtful teetotaler would have found abundant food for reflection in seeing a grave conclave of doctors tasting the beverage to see that it was properly compounded. I may add that it produced no evil effects among those who in every ward of the hospital afterward partook of it.

"Card playing, strictly forbidden in our hospitals, is rather encouraged in the hospitals here and the men gamble with impunity, their stakes being 'pfennig,' a coin equal to about one-third of a cent. A loss or gain which amounts in the course of an evening to two 'groschen' (five cents) is considered colossal. Only a single instance of insubordination requiring punishment has come to my knowledge, and not one occasion of a quarrel leading to violence. My purpose in citing these facts is to illustrate the temperance and moderation of the Prussian soldier, which enable him to venture safely upon ground which for us is fraught with danger.

"There is a distinction between Prussian sub-

jects of which you may not have heard: Stock
Preusse, and Muss Preusse. These expressions
appeared in the provinces which Prussia conquered and annexed in the wars of 1864–1866—
Hesse and Holstein, where there was at first dis-
affection. The Hessians and Holsteiners jeeringly
called the conquerors, for their stiff military bearing, 'Ramrod Prussians,' Stock Preusse; while
these in retaliation dubbed the Hessians and Holsteiners 'Have-to-be' Prussians, Muss-Preusse.
Today however, the formerly lukewarm Rhine-
landers, the indifferent Hessians, and Hanove-
rians, the disaffected Poles, the subjugated Holsteiners show no trace of disloyalty. Numerous
dwellers from these provinces have been in my
charge, and there are no indications of opposition
to the powers that be. There has of course been
dissatisfaction with the war, and murmuring at
individual hardship; but of this there was more
from the old Prussian Landwehrmen (who had
gone through '64 and '66, and been long away
from their homes) than among the new recruits,
elated by their first taste of glory and adventure,
under the victorious Prussian standard. Prussia
has won to herself by her victories the hearts of
her newer subjects.

"The visiting staff of our hospital is composed almost exclusively of private practitioners
of the city of Cassel, in contact with whom one

was able to see much of the average doctor of
medicine. The advantages which long discipline
and careful training confer upon the followers of
any vocation are apparent in the practice of every
physician observed here. In the United States,
graduation from Medical School is all that is required for establishing a practice; but here a
severe state examination must be passed before
practice can be undertaken. That ability is more
marked or talents greater than with Americans of
the same calling no one would claim, but that
talent can here be turned to better account no
one could deny. The German graduate in medicine is as a rule more firmly grounded, widely informed, and thoroughly drilled, than he of our
country, and for reasons which lie upon the surface of the educational systems of the two countries—or say, in the necessities of a new country
and the advantages of a long-established one.
Deliberation, learning, system, prudence are con-
spicuous in the performances of these men. They
have acquired the equivalent of a college degree
before beginning to study medicine. They are
familiar with the more advanced methods of investigation as well as with such treatment of
disease as the science and research of an older
country and civilization are making available today. A far larger proportion of these practitioners than with us are skilled in the use of the

microscope, while the ophthalmoscope and the laryngoscope which are now [1870] being introduced in the United States have been in use here for some years. As surgeons, the Germans must yield to us in ingenuity and practical skill, but their caution and thorough methods lead them to results perhaps more remarkable. In a sudden emergency, a very difficult and serious operation (ligation of the common carotid artery) was performed successfully in our hospital by an elderly practitioner who had scarcely employed a surgeon's knife for twenty years; the operation was far from brilliant, yet the manner in which the unexpected demand was met showed how well the foundations in anatomy had been laid; a life in the utmost danger was saved. Numerous instances of the same kind, but less striking, have occurred. In the prescribing of medicines and drugs, good sense and sagacity are shown by these men: only a small number of drugs of proved efficiency is used. The medium, not the largest, admissible dose of any given medicine is employed, and only when there is the clearest indication for its use. So-called 'shot-gun' prescriptions are less often used than with us.

"The management of apothecary shops and system of dispensing deserves a word of comment. If any question rises concerning a prescrip-

tion it is sent back to the doctor for correction or
confirmation before being filled. The precautions
taken against the incorrect compounding of drugs
are such that a fatal mistake is almost unheard
of. One must admit however, that there are
many old fogies and many who have hobbies, as
is found to be true everywhere, and it would be
no injustice to some of these phlegmatic doctors
to call them unenterprising. Many here who have
been brilliant at the Gymnasium and the University relapse into apathy in later life when the spur
of necessity is removed. While with us almost
everything depends upon the individual, here
perhaps too much depends upon the University
and upon a Government which regulates too
many details.

"In both Field and Reserve Hospitals, the
duties of the nurse have been largely in the hands
of the various Protestant and Roman Catholic
sisterhoods whose services have been placed at
the disposal of the military authorities by the
spiritual mother or dictatress. These devoted
daughters of the Church have followed close upon
the heels of the demon of war, and their min-
istrations and heroic labors during this memorable half year of carnage must be a subject of
deep admiration and gratitude to those who have
witnessed and shared in them."

I should like now to return with my reader to September of 1870 in France, to Pont à Mousson on the Moselle. The view of the town was pleasing in the extreme: its setting on the gleaming river, the church towers, the ancient stone bridge, the ruins of a castle on a vine-covered hill. What impressed me that September day in 1870 was the exhibition of the German armies in motion: a general forward movement was in progress toward Paris; thither the main thoroughfare led through Pont à Mousson, across the stone bridge which here spans the Moselle and was now supplemented by two pontoon bridges. All three were crowded with troops, foot and horse, artillery, ordnance, and supply trains. Every arm of the service was moving at double quick to concentrate for the beleaguering of the ill-fated capital; Paris was to suffer siege and bombardment through the coming winter. Infantry regiments marched in close ranks through the streets; artillery units, cavalry companies, followed each other in quick and colorful array. Very striking were the many-colored troops of cavalrymen— blue dragoons, Uhlans with long pennant-tipped lances, cuirassiers in white with steel breastplates, elaborately accoutered hussars. These, with artillerists, sappers, commissary squads, and trains, made a spectacle not to be forgotten.

It was an interesting, if not entirely happy,

experience, on first arriving in Pont à Mousson, to be quartered for the night in an attractive residence. The orderly having the matter in charge accompanied me. I was given a pleasant room and did not see any of the household until morning, when, descending to the ground floor, I encountered a fine-appearing woman. She came toward me, and said that coffee would be served at once. I expressed thanks but said I would have *déjeuner* at the hotel. The sad and troubled countenance of this woman made me decide to be no longer an intruder in this home of one of the conquered. I engaged a room over a shop on a street near the market place. One observed the reaction of the people to the conditions of enemy occupation. Carts or wagons loaded with sick and wounded, both French and German, often came through the streets; and when they halted, passers-by would gather round, pressing upon their compatriots tokens of good will, flowers, delicacies, words of sympathy; but these were proffered only to the French; indifferent or scornful looks were directed toward the detested "Allemand." Opposite the Moselle bridge a considerable eminence overlooked the town; it was surmounted by the ruins of a medieval castle, named Mousson, which had given to the town its name. Climbing the hill one day, I gained impressive views: on the south a peaceful valley, fields of grain, grazing flocks and herds; to the north, war-torn land, smoking ruins, hills where life-and-death struggle for possession had taken place— the fields of St. Privat and Gravelotte, where Marshall Bazaine (now shut up in Metz) was defeated with his army of one hundred and seventy thousand men. The battles fought in this region had been the turning-point of the war. Bazaine was never able to break the investment thrown around Metz, though he attempted a sortie, in preventing which the Germans lost three thousand men. In the end Metz capitulated, on October 27, when two thousand souls surrendered to hunger and bombardment.

Through the winter of 1870–71 my colleague Graham and I served in the reserve hospital in Hessen Cassel. We became familiar with the life of this provincial city and the surrounding country, ruled by Prussia since the war of 1866 and the Austrian defeat at Sadowa. Wilhelmshöhe, the former palatial residence of the old Elector of Hesse, was situated two or three miles out from the town and had been made the place of detention of Napoleon III. On my first Sunday in Hesse I visited this suburb with twofold interest: to see the emperor's prison and to view the famous "waterworks," then second only to those of Versailles. (This huge system of ornamental water display was constructed largely with the funds which Great Britain paid for the Hessian soldiers sold by the Elector to her for military service against the colonies in our Revolutionary War. Fifteen million dollars were paid for twenty-two thousand Hessians, hired out and transported to America.)

The palace stood out from the background of a lofty wooded ridge. Visitors were admitted to the courtyard, where a placid sheet of water reflected banks covered with shrubs and shaded by splendid trees. On the far side of the lake as we entered we saw Napoleon in civilian garb with some of his attendant suite. In movement and attitude he appeared somewhat inert and bowed. It had been announced that the *Wasser Sprünge* would play on this Sunday; and soon the floodgates of the great reservoir in the hills above were opened, and the cascades, the fountain, and the cataract began to pour out their wealth of waters. The grand fountain threw a column of water to a height of two hundred and eighteen feet; it emerged in the center of the lake in the palace court. It was then the highest artificial vertical column of water known in Europe. Looking upward from the palace court, we saw the great cascade, more than forty feet in width, which plunged from the octagon tower at the top of the hill, and, falling into a succession of basins for a distance of eight hundred feet, plunged into the "Neptune Reservoir" below. From the reservoir two streams emerged, one into the aqueduct, the other over rocks built of masonry in imitation of the falls of Tivoli. There was a "Devil's Bridge," and near it "Pluto's Cave," while an imitation feudal castle, the Loewenburg, with moat and drawbridge, completed this triumph of artificiality. The most astonishing feature of the whole system was the octagon tower which stood at the top of the lofty range of hills, where reservoirs held back the accumulated water for the weekly display; the tower was surmounted by a pyramid, upon which stood a bronze statue of Hercules, thirty-one feet in height. By climbing a winding stair from below, one could arrive in an observatory built in the base of Hercules' club! Here eight or nine persons could collect and could get a magnificent view of hills and valleys, the city of Cassel, and the Fulda River, a thousand feet below.

During the winter of 1870-71 the service took on a routine character. Great interest was aroused when, after its long grueling siege, Metz capitulated, and Marshall Bazaine, General Canrobert, and many of the French staff came to Cassel as paroled prisoners to visit their fallen chief. The hotel where these officers, once high in the decadent empire, were now nominal pris-

oners was the scene of much excitement. They had
brought with them, besides their showy uniforms,
much of military accouterment; and their dash-
ing equipages (some of which were later auctioned
off) attracted much attention. It was rumored that
Empress Eugénie had made a secret visit here to
her fallen consort.[3] Cassel had been the center of
the kingdom of Westphalia, created by Napoleon
I. It will be remembered that Napoleon annulled
the marriage of his brother Jerome to Miss Eliza-
beth Patterson, of Baltimore (though the pope
refused his sanction), and compelled Jerome to
marry the Princess of Württemberg, in 1807.
Here Jerome reigned for six years of extrava-
gance and misrule. There were still to be seen
landmarks of that "reign"—the Chateau, and
marble baths embellished with sculpture.

In April I received honorable discharge from
the service, and departed for Berlin, with the
double purpose of settling my account with the
government and of enrolling for special medical
study in the University. The government had
placed the affairs of the American volunteer surgeons in the hands of Friedrich Kapp, a German
historian, politician, and lawyer, who had lived in
New York for twenty years and had now returned

[3] The recently published letters of the Empress Dowager of Frederick
III to her mother Queen Victoria, in which she tells of this secret visit
of Eugénie to her husband, confirm what was at the time a rumor.

to reside in Germany. Graham and I called upon him; found him a very pleasant gentleman, and interested for our advantage. He gave us an introduction to Ludwig Bamberger, a member of Parliament (Bundesrath and Reichstag), which was then in session. Bamberger pointed out to us the crown prince, afterward Emperor Frederick III, General von Moltke, and other celebrities. Mr. Kapp secured for us, in addition to compensation for our services, an amount sufficient to meet the expenses of the return to America. The amount paid us monthly while we were in Cassel had been seventy-five thalers ($56.25 in American money); the Prussian government had a reputation for frugality.

Matriculating at the University of Berlin, I became a member of a special class in microscopy, conducted by the illustrious Professor Virchow, author of *Cellular Pathology*. Virchow was not only pre-eminent in medical science; he was an active liberal in politics, was a member of Parliament, and opposed Bismarck's absolutist policies. He had had the honor of being challenged to a duel by Bismarck; had refused to fight but had been earnestly besought by more than one student to allow the student to meet Bismarck in his stead. The spring and summer in Berlin were full of interests of many sorts. At the Charité

Hospital I saw mental patients, unaware that such patients were afterward to be my special charge; attended the surgical clinic of the famous Langenbeck, who demonstrated a series of amputations; also made the acquaintance of Professor Virchow, who was most kind and approachable. He was an indefatigable worker, commonly found in the evening bowed over his desk, which was so piled with accumulated papers as hardly to leave him room to write. Often we saw upon the streets generals who had won fame in the war just ended, statesmen and princes of the royal blood. The old Kaiser, Wilhelm I, almost daily sat at his desk in a window of the palace in Unter den Linden, seen by all passers-by and frequently responding to salutes. In May I heard Bismarck discuss the terms of the peace treaty later concluded at Frankfort (May 23, 1871); Bismarck was not a fluent speaker but was forcible through the qualities that gained for him his title, the "Iron Chancellor."

Of interest at this period to the nation, and especially to the world of music, was an event at which I happened to be present. I refer to the coming of Richard Wagner from Bayreuth, where he was then building his National Theater and Opera House, to Berlin, to direct a grand concert in the Berlin Opera House; on this occasion his

newly composed "Kaisermarsch" in honor of the
creation of the German Empire had its first presentation. The event was managed in true Wag-
nerian style; the program contained only Wagner's own compositions, with the exception of a
symphony of Beethoven; under his baton stood
and sat hundreds of singers and players of instruments. On this occasion he truly represented
musical imperialism and pomp—his back to an
audience unprecedented, of royalty, of the moment's great in civil and military power, in art.
A touch of humor was introduced by his immense
scarlet handkerchief, hanging from the pocket of
his "spike-tail" coat.

Another impressive event of these days was the
formal celebration of the victory over France, of
the recovery of the lost provinces, and the establishment of the German Empire under the he-
gemony of Prussia. This was commemorated for-
mally by the triumphal return of the army, and a
victorious entry, *Einzug*, into Berlin. Weeks
were spent in preparation for this event, which
occurred on June 16, 1871. A great scheme
of decoration and beautification of the city had
been carried out: gigantic groups of temporary
statuary were erected at the city gates and in
front of the imperial palace; festoons, flags, banners, wreaths, covered its walls. Unter den Lin-

den was lined with rows of captured cannon. Before the imperial palace was placed a colossal figure of Germania, seated, wearing a crown, with maiden figures, Alsace and Lorraine, at her side; molded in high relief upon the great pedestal were figures of heralds summoning the troops, warriors rallying to the call. At the Potsdam Gate, a winged Victory rose above a pyramid of captured cannon; the pedestal held the inscription "Sedan"; at her right and left stood figures representing Metz and Strassburg. At the Halle Gate towered "Berolina," with bruins at her feet. Other statues of Victory stood at the cross-streets; canvasses depicted Prussian victories.

On the morning of the sixteenth, one hundred and forty thousand troops gathered at their respective rallying-places and, marching forward, united at the Thiergarten Park, ready to pour through the Brandenburg Gate, into the Pariser Platz, thence into Unter den Linden. The stately embassies of foreign nations face the Pariser Platz: the English, the French, and the Russian (the French at that juncture showed no signs of life). Above towered the massive columns of the Brandenburg Gate, its summit surmounted by the "Quadriga of Victory," the chariot and horses of bronze, removed by the first Napoleon in 1807, and restored after his defeat. In the Platz, the vanguard of the triumphal procession made its appearance. The three greatest personalities of the war and of the state advanced abreast, mounted and in gala uniform: Bismarck, wearing steel helmet, white uniform, of his favorite Kurassier regiment; von Moltke, head of the general war staff; von Roon, minister of war, organizer of the army, and field marshal. The Kaiser came next, alone in his glory. At the Gate, seventy young women in white extended to him a welcome; farther on he halted to present a wreath to a group of crippled officers. A civil ceremony followed, in which Berlin's mayor and councilmen took part. The procession then moved forward, the crown prince and Prince Friedrich Karl with their staff officers followed by the rulers of Saxony, Bavaria, and other principalities. These were succeeded by the ladies of the royal families in open carriages, drawn by four-and-six-span teams, with coachmen, footmen, outriders, a series of splendid bouquets adorning the cavalcade. Then followed the troops, representing all branches of the service, marching to regimental music, with banners and trophies innumerable. Wreaths thrown from the side lines were caught on bayonets, grasped by eager hands. Each division was greeted with cheers by thousands

of eager spectators. And to the world was proclaimed the fall of Napoleon III, Prussia's recovery of "Elsass and Lotharingen," the creation of the German Empire. The day of triumph
was followed by a night of festivity: illumina-
tions, music, banqueting, revelry; gala performances in theaters and concert halls; reunions of
comrades in arms. Many danced and drank the
night away.

My course of study was finished; my thoughts
were turning homeward. Gladly I mapped my
return journey through Dresden, Prague, Nürn-
berg, down the Rhine to Cologne, thence via
Brussels to London. In London a pleasant re-
union with Graham occurred; he had left Germany after our discharge from the hospital service. We went to dinner with a London doctor
who served us grouse of his own shooting and a
variety of light and heavy wines, and who was
very hospitable. Though I had enjoyed in Germany the beer and wine which were a common
accompaniment, moderately indulged in, of all
food, I was revolted in London by the passion for
alcoholic stimulants everywhere in evidence. The
gin palaces were crowded by men and women, the
latter often with babies in their arms. I spent
two weeks in London, an eager sight-seer, and
heard memorable music at the Crystal Palace
and at Covent Garden.

In 1871 crossing to New York took thirteen days by the Inman Line. This was good time, considering we encountered a three-day gale which laid many of us low. Landing in New York on September 25, I found a letter offering a position in the State Hospital for Mental Diseases at Elgin, Illinois. Edwin A. Kilbourne, a classmate in the medical school, recently appointed medical superintendent of this hospital, wanted me as assistant.

The section of these reminiscences now to follow is a record of twenty-two years in the practice of psychiatry in the service of the state: eight as assistant in Elgin, and fourteen as medical superintendent of the new State Hospital at Kankakee, Illinois. At Kankakee a departure was made in construction of institutions for those afflicted with mental diseases; the institution there was the first in the United States to be built on the "cottage," or detached-ward, plan. During the fourteen years I spent as superintendent of this institution, it reached a capacity of two thousand patients; restraint had been abolished; a training school for attendants and nurses had been established; and a beginning had been made in occupational therapy. A political upheaval in Illinois in 1893 caused me to resign from my position at Kankakee. I then took charge of a sanitarium of my own at Wauwatosa, Wisconsin, the "Milwaukee Sanitarium," where I continued until my retirement in 1920 at the age of seventy-five.[4]

[4] [The author had planned to include in his autobiography an account of the years of his directorship of the Milwaukee Sanitarium—of which his successor, Dr. Rock Sleyster, is now in charge—and of the thirteen years spent in La Cañada, California, which followed. His death prevented the completion of the narrative.—EDITOR'S NOTE.]

CHAPTER THREE

The Years 1871-93

*Illinois Hospitals for the Insane: Jacksonville,
Elgin, Kankakee; Origin and Growth of the
Institution at Kankakee, Illinois;
Early Psychiatrists*

THE section of my book now beginning recounts the experiences by which I arrived at and carried forward my especial work in life. This came to be the care of people sick with mental and nervous diseases. It was coupled with the administration of institutions established for the care and treatment of such invalids. The effort for better conditions for men and women handicapped in life by these troubles was to be my vocation. During twenty-two years I was engaged in the institutions of the state, for twenty-five more in an institution of my own, and later, in private practice.

Arriving in New York from Germany in September, 1871, an unattached adventurer in the field of medicine, my cry was "Westward Ho!" This was the direction of thought and desire, for in the Midwest were family ties. The question before me now was that of making an entry into the practice of my profession, of getting launched on the wide ocean of medicine. I had found awaiting me in New York an offer of a position in the State Hospital for Mental Diseases at Elgin, Illinois. In part this offer influenced me.

On starting west, my first stop was Clinton, New York, where in Dwight's Rural School I had, as a youth from the age of twelve to fifteen, prepared for college; I now became a guest in the home of Dr. Dwight for a time. Some account has been given of the Rural High School, and of Rev. Benjamin W. Dwight, eminent educator and philologist, founder and headmaster of the school, first in Brooklyn and afterward in Clinton, New York. In an intellectual sense he had been a father to me; and at this time a nearer relationship was gained, for I became engaged to Lillian, his eldest daughter, now twenty-one. I had been enthralled by her beauty two years before, but had not declared myself until now.

While I was in Clinton, on October 9, 1871, word came of the great conflagration in Chicago, where the homes and places of business of one hundred thousand inhabitants had been swept from the face of the earth in a few hours' time. Two hundred and fifty lives were lost; one hundred thousand were rendered homeless. Four million dollars were given by the world in relief. (In this country only one greater fire has occurred, that in San Francisco following the earthquake in 1906.) A relative, Judge Elliot Anthony, who lived in Chicago, had been burned out of house and home. He possessed a valuable library, and in his anxiety to prevent its loss he took steps to save it. Knowing the conflagration was on its way, and calculating that he had an hour's leeway, he took the time to have men dig a pit in his front yard. In the bottom of this he laid carpets torn from the floors; then, piling his most valuable books on these, he had them covered with more carpets; the earth was shoveled back. But the effort was in vain; the fire reached the edges of the carpets, burrowed down into the pit, and destroyed all.

From Clinton I went to South Haven, a port on the shore of Lake Michigan; here my people were living, in a region of pine woods. Manufacture of lumber was the business of the place. A great stertorous sawmill was in operation, whose product of timbers and planks was sent across the lake to the Chicago market. In this sawmill I had, as already related, spent two summer vacations. I had operated the buzz saw, which performs two operations in one: taking the rough edge off planks and boards, and making a by-product, lath and siding. New mill hand as I was, I had on one occasion approached the saw without sufficient respect, and still carried on my left hand a slight scar as a reminder of those days. After the home greeting in South Haven, I went to Chicago to meet Dr. Kilbourne, from whom, on arriving in New York, I had found a letter, to discuss with him the question of a position in the new State Hospital for Mental Diseases at Elgin, Illinois, to which he had been appointed superintendent. I found Chicago still smoking in its ruins; the air was laden with the odor of parched wheat from a great smoldering grain elevator. A limited area on the West Side had escaped the conflagration, and here one could find lodging. I met my friend Kilbourne and learned more details about the position in question. The north wing of the building had been completed; it would accommodate three hundred patients and would be ready for occupancy in three months.

At this point I wish to go back to the period of my medical studies at the University of Michigan, from 1866 to 1869. I had graduated at Ann Arbor from the School of Medicine; but something I had not then realized now stared me in the face. This was my lack of preparation for practice in the care and treatment of mental patients. This deficiency in my case was not different from that of every man who graduated in that day from Ann Arbor or from any other of the medical schools in this country. Mental disease was not then, nor until long after, included in their curricula. Premedical studies were not then required in preparation for the course in medicine; I had had two years in arts and letters, but no courses in physics or chemistry, which were not then "prerequisite." The conditions that prevailed in 1866 deserve to be described by way of contrast to those of the present day, which still perhaps leave something to be desired. The Medical School at Ann Arbor was fully abreast of the best schools of the time; its courses of didactic lectures were thorough, and required six months, though the same subjects in many colleges were completed in but four. To obtain practical experience, the student in medicine rode with a preceptor between the courses. Ann Arbor was then a small college town, possessing neither hospital nor clinic. Students were obliged to go elsewhere for this training, as I had done after graduation. The courses in anatomy and physiology were conducted by the same professor, who also demonstrated the brain and cranial nerves; brain localization was in its rudimentary stage. Studies of Broca and Ferrier were coming to be known. Clinical cases in internal medicine and in surgery were occasionally presented in connection with the lectures. A good laboratory for analytical chemistry and for the elements of organic chemistry was maintained. There was no teacher of neurology, and the term "psychiatry" was unfamiliar. Nothing was taught concerning mental disease, then called "lunacy" or "insanity," a thing apart. The term "psychosis" might have been found in the dictionary but not in the current speech of students. In the twenty years after 1866, men could graduate in medicine without having seen a case of mental disease. Neurasthenia, sometimes called "Americanitis," had been described and named by Beard[1] in an article in the *Boston Medical and Surgical Journal* in 1869; but his book, *Practical Treatise on Nervous Exhaustion*, did not appear until 1880. Of textbooks on mental disease, I had seen none, to study them, until late in 1871, when I decided to go to the State Hospital. I then secured and read diligently such works as I could obtain.[2]

[1] Priority in naming and describing neurasthenia belongs to Van Deusen of Michigan State Hospital. He used the name and described the symptoms in February, 1869, in his hospital report, while Beard's first publication came out in April, 1869, and Beard's book did not appear until 1880. The facts are given by Bassoe in *Transactions of the American Neurological Association, 1927*. Neither Beard nor Van Deusen knew of the other's work.

[2] Bucknill and Tuke, *Manual of Psychological Medicine* (1858); Blandford, *Insanity and Its Treatment* (1871); Griesinger, *The Pathology and Therapeutics of Mental Diseases* (1845, translation); Maudsley, *Body and Mind* (1873); Griesinger, *Physiology and Pathology of Mind* (1876). The only American book was Hammond's *Diseases of the Nervous System* (1871). American textbooks which I had studied were: Isaac Ray, *Medical Jurisprudence of Insanity* (1838); Benjamin Rush, *Medical Inquiries and Observations upon Diseases of the Mind*. This last was out of print and could be found only in medical libraries. This was true also of *Treatment of Insanity* by John M. Galt, Jr. (1851).

Of instruments of precision, afterward universally in use, only the stethoscope was generally employed; the clinical thermometer was just becoming known; the ophthalmoscope had not come into general use, nor had the hypodermic needle or the laryngoscope, though these last had been known since the early fifties.

The offer which my friend Kilbourne was now making, of an appointment in the State Hospital, opened possibilities which I had never considered. Was I fitted for this special type of practice? I could not answer; but thus far I had not been attracted to any particular branch or specialty, and this unknown field had attractions. I was conscious of an interest in mental disease. I could recall portrayals in books—Ophelia, Hamlet, Lear, the Bride of Lammermoor, Jane Eyre, tales of mad regicides, King David's simulation, a woman I had encountered in the grounds of the Charité in Berlin. I decided to accept the position now offered by Kilbourne, who did not seem to be troubled by my lack of special preparation; and as the Hospital could not be opened for some months, I went in the meantime to the Central State Hospital for Insane at Jacksonville, Illinois, to acquire familiarity with my prospective duties. On Thanksgiving Day, 1871, Dr. Carriel, superintendent of the Central Hospital, invited me to become a guest member of his medical staff; and

from then until the following January, I was
occupied with study and practice in the care and
treatment of the hundreds of men and women
lost to the outside world by reason of mental
infirmities, who were now housed in this impressive, many-storied building provided by the
state. I began here the study of the derange-
ments and maladaptations denoted by the word
"insanity" which were to engage my efforts for
more than half a century, and still engage them.
Coming face to face with these fellow-beings,
doomed to separation from the outside world, I
realized that I had all to learn; my training in
school, in hospital, and in Germany had not provided me with an approach to the understanding
of these patients or of their special needs.

At that period, except for certain gross injuries
of the brain, the relationship between insanity
and the brain was not understood; such a relationship was believed to exist but had not been
proved. Disorders of the mind were held to be of
spiritual and intangible cause; and by the un-
lettered, to be associated with evil spirits and
with devils which must be "cast out." The principles upon which the origin of brain disease were
based and upon which it could be studied were
unknown, having only recently begun to be eluci-
dated. An epoch-making revelation of the source
of disease had only recently been made: one great

investigator of the nineteenth century, Rudolph Virchow, had by the publication of his book, *Cellular Pathology*, in 1858, given to the world the key to the organic origin of disease in the tissues and cells of the body. All living matter was now seen to be constructed of cells; the very fibers connecting one cell with another were revealed to be of cellular construction. It was now established as fact that the cell, that minute living structure visible only with the aid of the microscope, was the source of life and death, of life in health, and of death in disease. Heart, brain, bone, muscle—all were built of cells which differed in each organ but were homogeneous in each organ. It was found that the cells of the brain are the most complicated and difficult to study; brain anatomy was in its infancy.

In this new country, research and fundamental study of origins and causes of disease was not and could not be undertaken and carried through systematically as was possible in Europe. In the Old World, where an educated leisure class had grown up, many of whose members gave themselves to research and higher learning, such study was being prosecuted. In America the attention of the medical mind was absorbed by the necessities of general practice; the time for research and division of practice into specialties had not arrived. Now, in the light of *Cellular Pathology*, the brain and organs of the body were yielding their secrets. Studied under the microscope, lungs, liver, kidney, and nervous tissue showed change produced by disease; diseased cells were found which accounted for symptoms seen at the bedside. The brain, however, when examined microscopically, yielded at first no insight into mental changes (except in diseases like tumor, trauma, or hemorrhage, where motion was paralyzed and consciousness abolished). At that time if tissues of two brains, one of a normal subject and one of a case of pronounced mania, were placed under the microscope, no difference might be observed between them. Years of investigation were necessary to reveal the disease processes. Advances had to be made in finer adjustment of instruments, in staining the cells to make them visible, in sectioning them with delicate section-cutters; also in understanding chemical reactions of blood and lymph, the effect of internal glandular secretions, before more minute changes could be discovered and interpreted. Furthermore, mental mechanisms, reactions in thought and action, had to be studied and interpreted, in order that the whole should be co-ordinated and associated with mental syndromes. Virchow's discovery of the law, "Omnis cellula e cellula," had to be applied with the knowledge that every cell, diseased or healthy, came from another cell; that disease springs from injury to cells by toxic or mechanical agencies; that multiplication of healthy cells produces health, that of pathologic cells produces disease. *Cellular Pathology* taught the world this lesson and explained the mysteriousness of mental disease and the delay in research concerning it.

It may be stated here that there are two views of the question whether or not mental disease in its more subtle forms can be traced to, or identified with, diseased changes in the brain cells; to abnormal reactions in blood and fluids of the brain. The physiological school holds that it can; the psychological school studies consciousness and the subconscious only, without reference to the tissue of the brain. The psychoanalytical school, founded by Freud, maintains that physiological and medical knowledge is not requisite; that a Ph.D. can treat a psychoneurosis as well as an M.D. can treat it. This thesis has been maintained in a court of law in Vienna.[3]

In my first visits to the wards of the Jacksonville Hospital, seeing for the first time a large number of the mentally incapacitated, I was impressed with the infinite variety of ways in which mental integrity may be lost or impaired. The only condition that was common to all the pa-

[3] "Correspondence," *American Journal of Psychiatry*, November, 1931, p. 575.

tients was their compulsory sequestration. A general distinction was held between "front" and "back" wards: in the former were the quiet, the tidy, the industrious, the mild; in the latter the disturbed, the untidy, the obstreperous, the imbecile. These divisions presented many contrasts, mental and physical, a variety of defects and excesses in thought and action: outward-seeming normality and extreme eccentricity; inertia and elation; irritability and indifference; there were the blasphemous and the pious; the gay and melancholy; the mute and the garrulous; the genial and surly; victims of dementia praecox and of senility.[4]

Here was a domain which might be likened to some foreign country, whose inhabitants had manners and customs of their own. Some, without the common impulse of self-preservation, showed a strange ill will toward themselves, and had to be guarded from self-injury. Some were obsessed by strange visions; some, deaf to the outer world, heard mysterious voices; some suffered (or rejoiced) in loss of memory. They were alike only in each being different from the normal and from each other. Natural sights and sounds are perverted by disordered minds into words and im-

[4] Of 263,000 patients in state hospitals for mental disease in 1927, 114,240 were cases of dementia praecox, or schizophrenia; 13,585 were cases of senile dementia.

ages, creating illusions. Imagined sights and sounds, which have no basis in the outer world, are termed "hallucinations." Delusions differ from both; these are false ideas growing from disease of the mind, and fall into two classes: the wholly impossible and the systematized, or partially reasoned. Patients who manifest the latter are known as paranoiacs; they often hold a single, permanently fixed idea. Patients so afflicted are incurable. They often become unmanageable, fancying themselves wronged or persecuted and attacking others in revenge or in imagined self-defense; they are the more dangerous because they can reason on subjects other than that of their one delusion; hence their insanity may not be recognized until after a crime has been committed.

At Jacksonville I had my first experience with patients suffering from the disorders just described; here also I first encountered the various conditions resulting from amnesia, brain concussion, impaired consciousness, and other ills, then still unnamed. Just at this time at this hospital and among interested groups throughout the state there was much discussion caused by a crusade which a former inmate was carrying on. Mrs. E. P. W. had been confined as a patient in the institution for three years. Recently, upon obtaining her release, she had loudly proclaimed her wrongs; insisted that she had always been sound mentally; had been kidnapped and illegally confined. She attracted a good deal of attention, and a brief account of her story may here be set down as of interest in itself and because of consequences growing from it.

Whether at any time insane or not, Mrs. E. P. W. was now a woman of fine appearance, having shrewdness and ability. She spoke fairly well, and in parts of the state had attracted sympathetic attention. She had raised money by the sale of a pamphlet in which she described her wrongs; had appeared before legislative committees and enlisted champions of her cause among the lawmakers. Her history was briefly as follows: She had married a Presbyterian clergyman, pastor of a Congregational church in an Illinois village. Question as to her mental integrity had come about in this way: Her husband had invited her to take charge of the Bible class, which was languishing; she agreed and entered upon this duty. To make the class hour more interesting, she had introduced discussion of doctrinal points in Calvinistic theology—total depravity, freedom of the will, God's immutability, and like subjects. Interest was aroused and increased rapidly; the membership of the class grew from a handful to forty-six members; it no longer languished, but heterodoxy made its appearance;

heretical opinions were advanced; heated discussions on foreordination and predestination took place. Visions of discord, danger to orthodoxy, and possible disruption of the church began to obsess the deacons. It was felt the retirement of the class leader should be secured to avert disaster. The successful leader of the class refused to take this view; she took the position that her husband, having appointed her as leader of the Bible class, must either support her or forbid her further activity. She waited for him to act; and as he did nothing, she took occasion, on a Sunday when service was in progress and her husband in the pulpit, to enter the church, interrupt the proceedings, and demand a letter of dismissal from the deacons. Her conduct at this time produced the impression that she was insane; the majority of the villagers thought her so. In the course of time it was planned to take her to the state hospital; the sheriff took her to the railway station, but she refused to board the train. Seeing that compulsion would be used, she suggested that two men among the crowd collected to see her off should clasp hands to form a "saddle seat," and she would thus enter the train. Though she protested against the violation of her personal freedom, and insisted she did not go either of her own accord or by due process of law, she was taken to the state hospital and was there detained.

The warrant for her detention was the request of her husband, together with the approval of the medical officer in charge. Supposedly she had been lawfully held; but in reality her detention had been illegal, with consequences which I shall relate. The illegality arose from the following circumstances: There was an unconstitutional clause in the statute for commitment to the hospital; it had been for fourteen years on the books without having been questioned. This clause permitted a husband to certify that his wife was insane and, with the agreement of the doctor in charge of the hospital, to have her there confined. It is evident that Mrs. E. P. W. had never been lawfully committed; her liberty had been taken away without "due process of law"; and heavy penalties are the price of violation of this principle. Mrs. E. P. W. was a victim of kidnapping and of false imprisonment. A day of reckoning was at hand; and when it came, the husband was denounced and the doctor forced to resign his position. A sentiment in favor of Mrs. E. P. W. had been created throughout the state, and she was able to enlist the support of legislators at Springfield. As a result, the Jury Commitment Law was passed by the Illinois legislature in 1867. Owing partly to the same influence, similar laws were passed in Massachusetts and Iowa.

The Jury Commitment Law required that a

public hearing be instituted in each case of mental disorder before a patient could be sent to an institution. The result of the law was that patients and their friends or families would endure any hardship or suffering rather than take anyone they loved into court, to be publicly brought before a jury, pronounced insane, and so registered. For twenty-six years this law remained on the statute books despite efforts to repeal it. Because of it, hundreds of patients who ought to have gone to the hospital did not go, or went only when their cases had become chronic or hopeless.

Before giving an account of my return to Elgin and of my work there and at Kankakee, I shall consider briefly the advance in the nineteenth century in the care of the insane and the development of a humane attitude toward those so afflicted. In the early decades of the century, insanity was considered a hopeless condition; a man or brother so afflicted was lost to his natural world, was supposed to have no appreciation of kindness, no resentment of the reverse, to be destitute of feeling. He was looked upon with dread and repulsion, which attitude often bred thoughts of persecution. Finally the afflicted one might have to be confined under lock and key, and in that time hospitals for mental disease humanely managed did not exist.

In every movement for social reform, there are

always a few men or women who show more actively than others a zeal or genius for betterment. In the attitude toward insanity and in the field of psychiatry, two such men stood out at the end of the eighteenth century who, by their humanity and creative genius, initiated reforms which continued through the nineteenth century and are still inspiring in the twentieth. These men were Philippe Pinel, in France, and William Tuke, in England. Pinel in 1793 was given charge of Le Bicêtre with its two thousand inmates—criminals, paupers, and insane persons; the insane were chained in cells. The records showed that certain ones had been so confined for ten, for thirty-six, even for forty years, this treatment being administered at the discretion of a "keeper," who was ignorant and sometimes brutal. Pinel decided upon a policy of systematic removal of these instruments. In severe irony he declared the chains were "an admirable invention for perpetuating the rage of the maniac, and keeping in his heart an intensified desire to revenge himself."[5]

Cure of the patient could not be thought of under such conditions; but in the public mind of that period the only purpose for the existence of the asylum was confinement of dangerous per-

[5] *Les grands alienists français*, by Dr. René Semelaigne (Paris: Steinheil, Editeur), p. 73.

sons. The insane were not then believed to be "possessed of devils," but it was supposed that all insane persons must be dangerous. It was not realized that many were made dangerous by the treatment they received. None but the most benevolent had thought of treatment for the restoration of sanity; the treatment given was limited to bleeding, purging, cold showers, emetics. It was thought even by doctors that a shock might restore reason; frightening the patient was at times recommended, letting him think he was to be killed, or plunging him in cold water.

Pinel's appointment to the Bicêtre in 1793 happened in the midst of the Reign of Terror during the French Revolution. Pinel was a republican, but an enemy of the outrages committed in the name of reform. He had been obliged, as a member of the guard, to witness the guillotining of Louis XVI.[6] His position in the Bicêtre was under the authority of the Commune, and to carry out his ideas of reform he must have the approval of the central powers. The president of the Commune, Couthon, an ally of Robespierre, was suspicious of Pinel's request, and roughly addressed him: "Bad luck to you, Citizen, if you are deceiving us, and if among your foolish ones in the asylum you are concealing enemies of the people." Pinel replied that what

[6] Biography of Pinel by his nephew.

he was proposing was his plan as a physician for the good of his patients. Couthon, still suspicious, had himself transported next day to the asylum. On being taken to the quarters of patients chained in their cells, Couthon was impressed; he attempted to question the madmen, but received only insults in reply. Turning to Pinel, he exclaimed: "Citizen, are you not yourself a fool to wish to unchain such animals?" Pinel replied: "I am convinced that it is only because these men are deprived of air and liberty that they are intractable." Couthon answered: "Do what you wish; but I fear you will become the victim of your presumption." Couthon took his departure, and on the same day Pinel began the reforms upon which he had decided. He released a few of the patients. One, an English officer, a prisoner for years, when led into the sunlight, cried "Ah, que c'est bon!" After his release he remained quiet, and after two years was given his liberty. Another, a victim of religious mania, had become a complete cripple and died soon after.[7] To one ten years in manacles, Pinel remarked: "Give me your hand. You are reasonable; I am going to employ you."[8] Pinel had

[7] Semelaigne, *op. cit.*

[8] This was Chévigne, who had been confined ten years in the Bicêtre. He was employed by Pinel, and later saved the life of Pinel from a mob who accused him of having protected royalists in the Bicêtre.

made himself familiar, by frequent visits, with the personality of each of the patients he now liberated; he had, moreover, in the person of a lay assistant, Pussin, long in service at the Bicêtre, an invaluable aid.

It was shortly demonstrated that there was no danger, but rather benefit, from this deliverance. The achievement of Pinel became known, and his example was followed in other countries. In France he came to be known as "Le Bienfaiteur des Alienés"; a statue was erected in his honor by the Société Medico-Psychologique of France[9] in 1885, the statue being appropriately placed in the Place de la Salpêtrière.

Scarcely less than Pinel's renown in France was the fame achieved in England by William Tuke, a merchant of York, the originator of the York Retreat. He was a man of great benevolence of character, a Quaker, and became convinced from personal experience that existing institutions, with their methods of force and use of restraint by means of straight-jackets, leather muffs, belts, even chains, were conducted on wrong principles. With this conviction he determined to bring into existence an institution of a different character, which should exemplify the religious principles of the Society of Friends. He called a meeting of his co-religionists and organized a successful

[9] René Semelaigne, *op. cit.*

movement; collected funds; had plans made for a building; and in 1776 a central block with two wings was completed. Thus the York Retreat was established and became famous in the annals of psychiatry. Here kindness was the rule of conduct; and the more mild, intelligent, and humanitarian animating spirit seemed to call forth a response of similar attitude from the patients. Every means at hand of diverting thought and action from morbid into healthful channels and of furnishing natural exercise and employment was brought into use. These methods were found to be beneficial, even curative, and won approval wherever known; through them the fame of the York Retreat was established. For four generations the Tuke family enjoyed high reputation in their profession. Henry Tuke, son of William; Samuel, son of Henry; and Daniel Hack Tuke, son of Samuel, in succeeding generations, from 1796 to 1885, added to the family renown. Samuel Tuke wrote a book describing the York Retreat,[10] which made it widely known. The Frankford Retreat in Pennsylvania, opened in 1817, was modeled upon Samuel Tuke's description of the York Retreat.

In the early decades of the nineteenth century adequate care of sufferers from mental disease did

---

[10] *Description of the York Retreat* (1813); translated into German by Jacobi of Sieberg, Nestor of German alienists.

not exist except in some rare, favored spot like the York Retreat. In France, notwithstanding the example of Pinel, the insane were immured with criminals and paupers in prisons and work-houses until in 1838,[11] a plan for state care reached completion. In England the conditions in the London Asylum Bethlehem (corrupted to "Bedlam") were so bad that they led to public scandal and a Parliamentary investigation. It was found that patients were exhibited to the jeering public for a fee; many were confined in cells; medical care consisted in blood-letting, purging, use of emetics, and fasting. Straight jackets, leather muffs, and belts were in frequent use. When these conditions were exposed, a strong public sentiment for reform was aroused; and when in 1839 Dr. John Conolly, a London physician whose name should follow those of Pinel and Tuke, inaugurated a movement for abolishing all mechanical restraint, his efforts met with strong public support. He (Conolly) was placed in charge of the great London Asylum at Hanwell, and there abolished every form of mechanical restraint. No device of this kind was permitted in the establishment. Legislation was ultimately adopted which forbade the use of restraint except in extreme cases. In 1877 Lord Shaftesbury, chief of the Commissioners in

[11] *Encyclopaedia Brittanica*, XII 390.

Lunacy, stated in a Blue Book: "Mechanical restraint has been abolished in every asylum in
the country."[12]

The following quotation from the writings of
John Conolly shows the sincerity and benevolence which animated him: "None but those who
live amongst the insane can fully know the pleas-
ures which arise from imparting trifling satisfac-
tions to impaired minds. None else can appreci-
ate the reward of seeing reason returning to a
mind long deprived of it."[13]

In modern times in our own country there was
an era of indifference. When the Civil War was
at an end, it was found that the number of those
afflicted with mental disease had greatly increased. Almshouses and jails, where meager
shelter was grudgingly provided by town or
county, were the only resort for the throngs of
human derelicts. Gradually it was realized that
the state must assume the burden. At first the
only concern in the public mind was the provision
of custody; curative treatment was not thought
of as a possibility. Ultimately it became clear
that medical care was needed and that medical
men should have charge of these unfortunates.
In the later nineteenth century the influence of

[12] W. Lander Lindsey, M.D., F.R.S.E., "Mechanical Restraint in
British Asylums," *American Journal of Insanity*, XXXV, 555 ff.

[13] Bedford Pierce (ed.), *Address to Mental Nurses* (London: Balliere
Tyndall & Cox, 1924).

philanthropy inspired the public mind; the "asylum" idea gave way to the "hospital" concept; the institution at Jacksonville was itself the outgrowth of the philanthropic energy and devotion of a single individual, Dorothea Dix.[14]

The reform work of Dorothea Lynde Dix began when, having been the successful head mistress of a school in Boston, she was invited to teach a class of girl convicts in the Massachusetts House of Correction. In meeting and teaching these unfortunate women, she acquired a knowledge of conditions in the institution—overcrowding, uncleanliness, the herding of the innocent with the guilty—conditions which at that time characterized prisons throughout the world. Her first step was an effort for the relief of a few insane women prisoners confined in bitterly cold rooms. She urged the official in charge to provide sufficient heat; but meeting with a refusal, she appealed to the judge, then conducting a trial in the adjacent courtroom. From him she obtained an order requiring the keeper of the prison to supply heat. Her greatest achievements were those which she perseveringly wrought for sufferers from mental disease. The results she attained were the outcome of the irresistible force she

[14] The account of Miss Dix is taken from Hurd's *Institutional History*, Vol. I, chap. iii, pp. 101 ff., made by Dr. Hurd from the biography by Tiffany and a paper by Dr. C. W. Page of Hartford.

exercised by her plan of campaign. She visited throughout the United States the haunts of misery—poorhouses and jails—where those of lost mentality had fallen. Of the very existence of the inmates the world at large was ignorant. She found them helpless, neglected, confined in degradation and filth. When the legislature of the state in question was in session, she brought these conditions in all their repulsiveness to the attention of the complacent and respectable law-makers. Her method was effective; her arguments irresistible. More than thirty institutions were created, altered, or enlarged in capacity as a result of her efforts. Not only in the United States and Canada, but in Great Britain, Germany, and France, Miss Dix prosecuted her benevolent work. At the Trenton Hospital, where by official invitation she spent her declining years, I visited her in 1876. She was then in her seventy-second year, frail physically but in undiminished mental vigor.

By slow and laborious stages the state has intervened. "The insane are wards of the state" is a saying attributed to Horace Mann. But even now, not one of the states of the Union supports all of its dependent insane; and great variation do the state institutions show: some are honestly administered; others are honeycombed with political corruption; in others there is political dry rot.

The achievement of Julia Lathrop, member of the Illinois State Board of Charities from 1893 to 1909, was significant. She, too, traveled upon miserable roads to visit remote county farms, almshouses, and asylums, where the insane were housed. She made known the conditions she found and then, though opposed at every step, began the leadership of a movement to have the insane transferred from county wardship to state institutions where scientific and efficient methods of treatment were being developed.

The Mental Hygiene movement, inaugurated by Clifford Beers, author of *The Mind That Found Itself*, began in 1908 in Connecticut, where Mr. Beers organized the first Mental Hygiene Society. In 1909 the National Committee of Mental Hygiene was created in New York, with Mr. Beers as secretary; in 1918 the Canadian Committee was organized. The first International Congress on Mental Hygiene held in Washington in May, 1930, passed successfully into history; in it more than fifty nations participated. There is not in the annals of psychiatry a more notable achievement than this of the author of *The Mind That Found Itself*. In results and purposes, it transcends the achievements of the earlier reformers; its scope is incomparably broader by reason of modern progress in science and because of the genius and resourcefulness of Clifford Withington Beers.

In January, 1872, preparation for the formal opening of the new State Hospital at Elgin, Illinois, led to my taking up my abode in that pleasant little city on the banks of the Fox River, thirty miles from Chicago. I found there a former Ann Arbor classmate, into whose home I was temporarily introduced.

It was necessary to arrange for a legislative visit, or junket, to the new Hospital. In addition to the legislators who came on the day of opening, there were: Governor John L. Palmer; Joseph Medill, of the *Chicago Tribune;* the board of three trustees of the Hospital—Mr. C. N. Holden, of Chicago, president; Dr. Oliver Everett, of Dixon; and Mr. Henry Sherman, the resident trustee— Colonel Shipman, the architect, a Civil War hero; and Dr. Edwin A. Kilbourne, my chief, the medical superintendent. These, with the legislative contingent and many local dignitaries, inspected the new buildings and partook of the dinner which put the great kitchen of the Hospital to its first use. There were speeches by Governor Palmer and Joseph Medill, congratulations and prophecies. After this formality was over, some little time was required for assembling the necessary force of domestic help, attendants, nurses, also for purchasing equipment, before we could be ready to receive the patients, of whom there was a waiting-list, a large number to be sent from the other overcrowded institutions of the state.

It was a winter of severe cold and abundant snow. "Uncle" Henry Sherman, the local trustee, with his lively team of chestnut horses, with their tinkling sleigh bells, and his roomy sleigh, often carried us to and from the institution. In May we began to receive the people for whose care and restoration our efforts were to be expended. For many, restoration was out of the question; our task for them would be to render their existence as tolerable as possible, not losing sight of any means available for their mental or physical betterment.

A serious difficulty presented itself as the wards began to fill. The prime necessity of water—for domestic use, for baths, steam, flushing the waste pipes—became embarrassing, as the supply which had been supposed ample from springs in the gravel hills above us proved inadequate. One of the first undertakings was the laying of water mains to the Fox River, an eighth of a mile away, to obtain a sure source of supply. No question obtruded as to the sanitary state of the water; the country about was sparsely settled, and in that day the Bacillus typhosus had not been discovered.

Among the patients who now soon filled the wards to capacity, I found much of interest, from both personal and professional standpoints. Of those received, the majority had been for years under care at the Central Hospital, at the Cook County Asylum, or in some private institution. For most, the hope of recovery could scarcely be entertained: for these little could be done beyond regulation of their sleep and food, attention to their minor ailments, providing some normal activity. There were a few whose illness was of recent origin, and whose prospect was therefore more favorable. There was the satisfaction of seeing some of these return in health and vigor to a useful life.

Studying the life-histories, so far as obtainable, of this large body of patients, I sought to arrive at some conception of the conditions precedent to the development of their malady. Certain antecedents and concomitants stood out in the life-history of very many. Inquiry was made as to the existence of mental disease in other members of the family. It was traceable in an eighth part of each one hundred of those whose history was obtainable. Thus, for about 12 per cent, heredity could be set down as a partial cause of their condition. To this it is probable that another 12 per cent would have been added had all the facts been known; for about one-half, no information could be obtained. (The existence of mental disease in one member of a family is commonly regarded as having more significance than is warranted; for where one member is affected, there are, on an average, three who escape.) Excessive use of alcohol is, directly or indirectly, a concomitant in about 15 per cent of the cases of mental disease, whose genesis is to be attributed to heredity and environment operating together. The victim of a hereditary handicap will often escape a collapse if external conditions of competence, comfort, and contentment prevail in his environment; where, however, an inherent constitutional weakness and instability are already present, a crisis in external affairs may cause a breakdown.

There was little in the life at Elgin that could interest the world outside. The patients who came and went—to their homes or to the life beyond—had interest for their doctor and nurse and their own people. Occasionally some striking personality drifted in, like the beautiful white-haired woman, whose career had been among the fortunate of the earth and who was now rendered tragic and despairing by a delusion that a fatal transformation was taking place in her body whereby she was to be changed into a creeping

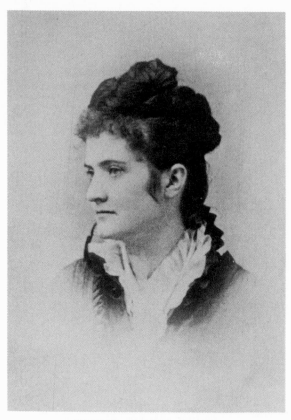

LILLIAN DWIGHT DEWEY

monster. To me, her doctor, she dilated upon the evidence that the dreaded transformation was taking place; that her arms were twisting backward, her head changing shape. When the governor of the state, John L. Beveridge, came to the Hospital, she requested an interview, and when it took place, requested that an order be issued by him that she should not be exhibited publicly when the loathsome transformation had taken place. Her health gradually failed. In her last hours she was still the victim of this delusion.

In January, 1873, I was married to Lillian Dwight, of Clinton, New York. We made our home in the Hospital at Elgin until 1879, when we moved to Kankakee, to the new hospital of which I was superintendent. There, in 1880, she passed to the life beyond. She had been a true and beautiful helpmeet.

During the years of my service at Elgin (1872–79), I studied with deep interest the local and national situation with regard to state policy for care of mental disease. I wrote and published a paper entitled, "Differentiation in Institutions for the Insane," advocating separate institutions for the epileptic, the alcoholic, and criminal cases, all of which were then found undifferentiated in each institution. I wrote also two papers entitled, respectively, "Present and Prospective Need of

Provision for the Insane" and "Provision for the Convict Insane." Rev. Frederick Howard Wines, secretary and moving-spirit of the State Board of Charities, and originator of the plan for detached wards or cottages in the construction of institutions for care of the insane, frequently discussed with me his profound conviction as to more homelike, less formal, and less expensive building-design. There were then hundreds of patients in the state of Illinois, in county almshouses and even in jails, not to mention those in private care, unprovided for. It might be supposed that those who were cared for at home were well situated; but experience had shown that the many were not, for ignorance and superstition sometimes prevented the provision of anything better than an unwholesome pen or cage. The problem was known, and its solution was a pressing matter in every state of the Union east of the Mississippi Valley; it existed also in the newer western states.

There was question of economy as well as of humanity; the institutions built thus far had ranged in cost from $1,000 per capita (this being the minimum) to $3,000 or $4,000. In the state of New York, at Poughkeepsie and at Buffalo, extravagant appropriations had been made. The corruption then prevailing under the Tweed régime in the city had extended to the state legislature. The cost per capita at Poughkeepsie and at Buffalo was $3,000 or $4,000 for each patient.[15] At that rate, the cost for each one thousand patients would come to $3,000,000 or $4,000,000, whereas a minimum of $1,000,000 for each thousand patients had been estimated. However, at that period (1870) $1,000,000 would accomplish more than would $3,000,000 at the present day (1930). Regarding the cost of buildings, it should be added here that a noteworthy demonstration of less expensive construction had been made in the additions to the Willard State Asylum, at Ovid, New York, by Dr. John C. Chapin, who had erected substantial buildings (in the old congregate style) at a cost of $500 per capita. Less expensive construction was retarded not only by the cupidity of the "grafter" but by the ordinary legislator's propensity to favor large appropriations which would minister to local pride in the erection of an institution stately and ornate in style of architecture. A central building of palatial style was considered necessary for the public offices, with spacious apartments in which the officers would reside. More thought was given to these features by most of the public officials than to the quarters intended for the mentally incapacitated. It was not supposed that

[15] Comments were made upon the magnificent buildings at Buffalo and at Poughkeepsie, the former with its twin ornamental towers estimated to have cost $70,000; also upon the grand ornamental double flights of stairs.

these humble individuals with darkened intellects were at all exacting or their requirements worthy of consideration. The institution, on the other hand, as befitting the dignity of the state, must be rendered imposing. The situation growing out of the love of display in the average legislator, supplemented by local pride and the sordid motives of the public plunderer, produced a state of affairs in which those who had at heart the welfare of the hundreds of insane, waiting in almshouses and jails, were faced by a well-nigh hopeless task. The general public was largely unaware or indifferent, having no conception of these unfortunates, increasing in every state of the Union. Two undertakings challenged the benevolent-minded few: first the public must be enlightened; then the cost of institutions must be reduced by half.

There were in certain of the states a few earnest and influential men and women who were alive to the situation: Members of the boards of commissioners of public charities in Massachusetts, New York, Ohio, Illinois (the only boards of charities then in existence), were aware of the difficulties and ready to grapple with them and with the politicians, who thought of the institutions mainly as of places for political favorites and protégés. Among the benevolent-minded in Illinois, one man stood out as possessing the intelligence

and force of character for dealing in a competent
and constructive manner with the situation.
This man was Rev. Frederick Howard Wines,
whom I have already mentioned, secretary of the
State Board of Public Charities at Springfield.
All who knew him were impressed by his genial
bearing, high principles, intellectual force, ability, and power of convincing speech. Furthermore, he had a conception and grasp of economic
detail unusual in a clergyman. Among his gifts
was that of being able to tell a story in a captivat-
ing way. In the late sixties the state legislature
had passed a law creating a State Board of Commissioners of Public Charities; the Board had
been appointed by Governor Palmer, and the
Governor had recommended the appointment of
Frederick Wines as secretary; it was a case of the
office seeking the man.

At this time, all matters relating to the care of
the mentally diseased in the United States, and
to the construction and control of state institutions for their accommodation, were strongly influenced and guided by the venerable organization, formed in 1844, the Association of Medical
Superintendents of American Institutions for the
Insane. This Association had formulated a body
of propositions regarding buildings, which had
been held, like the laws of the Medes and the
Persians, inviolable; they described in detail the

requirements considered by the Association necessary for all such structures. These, in brief, were to follow a certain uniform plan, to wit: a central structure for offices and residence of officers, with wings for the patients extending to right and left, usually four stories in height, with metal bars fixed in every window, exit and entrance controlled by a key in the hand of an attendant or keeper.[16] These institutions were described by the critical as prison-like in appearance.

It became more evident that this uniform design was being applied to multiform persons and conditions; the contrasts seen in the "front" and "back" wards were proof of this. And now, as opposed to the congregate structure just described (in 1880 the only type known in the United States), an idea representing reduction in cost, segregation, an entirely new type of construction, seemed to have taken possession of many minds; a construction resembling an ordinary house or home seemed to have its appeal.

[16] Illustrating what these locked doors and window bars meant to the patients, I quote remarks of some who were moved later to the new type of building, more like common dwellings. One said: "It is worth a dollar a day to go and come without asking someone to unlock the door." Another said: "It is just like being at home." Still another: "Putting my foot again right away on the ground is the biggest satisfaction I've known for years." It is unquestionable that the construction of "detached wards" by the new plan led immediately to greater freedom for the more quiet and trustworthy patients.

Cottage plan or detached ward expressed this new idea. The conservatives, as was to be expected, opposed the plan and used these terms in derision. In answer, instances were called to mind of provision for insane in foreign countries, where more simple, inexpensive construction prevailed, and investigation of which proved that the simpler construction had been less costly by half than that in the United States. This was true of colonies in France, of "open houses" in England, and of the village of Ghael in Belgium, where two thousand mental patients lived, most of them housed with the peasants; it was true also of a community in Scotland, where the patients were boarded out in the families of the farmers. By contrast, in the United States we had this inflexible plan for all the varying classes of patients, acute and chronic, quiet and disturbed, able-bodied and infirm, alert and impassive, industrious and idle. A call was beginning to be heard among the laity for more modern plans of buildings, for a departure from that structure inherited from the distant past—monastic, prison-like—upon which, as a model, thirty or more state institutions had been built. This "Kirkbride" plan, originally adopted by Dr. Thomas Kirkbride for the Pennsylvania Hospital, had been improved in detail and developed by the labors of successive physicians, architects, and humanitarians, notably by its originator, who was a man of excellent qualities, and to whom all honor is due. It was a plan, however, originally intended for acute cases, two hundred and fifty at most; had been adapted to care for six hundred, and finally for one thousand; and had been outgrown during the accumulation in the several states, through a score of years, of thousands of chronic and other cases, presenting all the forms of mental alienation. Institutions which would accommodate thousands had now to be provided.

Frederick H. Wines, acting as advisor of the Illinois State Board, urged the departure from the old plan of building. Two new institutions had been provided for by the Illinois legislature in the early seventies; and while they were building, he argued with the trustees, urging them so to vary the plans as to provide for even one small detached ward as an experiment; but these men could not see their way to departure from the established methods. When, however, in 1879, the law providing for the new hospital at Kankakee was passed, a clause was inserted making the approval of Frederick H. Wines and his Board obligatory in drawing up the plans. He was thus given his opportunity.

In the meantime the appointment in 1879 of myself as medical superintendent of the Kanka-

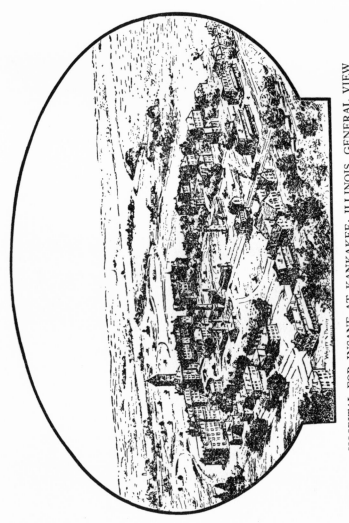

HOSPITAL FOR INSANE AT KANKAKEE: ILLINOIS, GENERAL VIEW

kee institution had occurred, and it therefore became my duty to work with Mr. Wines in this new departure. We planned the first detached wards, three buildings for one hundred patients, the middle one having a dining-room for all. These buildings fronted upon the south avenue laid out as a village street. According to the plan of Mr. Wines, an area of one thousand square feet was embraced in the plan, each of the four sides to form a street. On the east side, toward the Kankakee River, stood the main building, in the old style (the Board felt it necessary to yield thus far to the old policy, not to embark too rashly on an untried project). The north and south avenues were to be lined with cottage wards; a part of the west side and the center of the square were for service buildings.

Thus a beginning was made; and it is necessary only to add that the plan was carried on to completion, with general favor, so that at the next session of the legislature, appropriation was made of $400,000 to provide additional wards on the new plan for one thousand patients. Extensions were made from year to year until, when I retired in 1893, after fourteen years as medical superintendent, the four avenues had been entirely built up and the number of patients exceeded two thousand.

As showing the somewhat far-reaching influ-

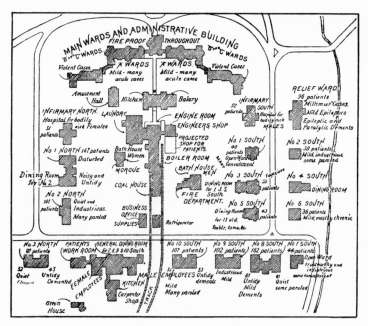

HOSPITAL FOR INSANE AT KANKAKEE, ILLINOIS
GROUND PLAN[17]

[17] In 1887, capacity, 1,600 patients; per capita cost, exclusive of running expense, $754.50; construction alone, $590.18.

ence of the experiment at Kankakee, the following facts may be noted: During the year 1883 the governors of Ohio and Indiana, each accompanied by a state commission and an architect or engineer, visited and inspected our institution. Later the institutions at Toledo, Ohio (capacity, one thousand), at Logansport, Indiana (capacity, three hundred and eighty), and at Richmond, Indiana (capacity, four hundred), were constructed on the new plan. North Dakota employed Major Willett, architect of the Kankakee Hospital, and in 1885 had provision for one hundred and sixty patients in three ward buildings. New York constructed a new hospital at Ogdensburg on the new plan in 1890, with capacity, when complete, of fifteen hundred patients. Ontario had in 1890, at Mimico near Toronto, detached wards for two hundred and forty. New York City in 1889 had three hundred and sixty patients in detached wards at Central Islip.[18] Freedom in construction then resulted from the experience at Kankakee; the change would have

[18] Anyone interested in the views on building plans in that period can find documents and discussions in the files of the *American Journal of Insanity* and in the *Propositions and Resolutions* collected and published in 1876 by the Association of Superintendents; also the reports of the Boards of Public Charities of New York, Massachusetts, Pennsylvania, and Illinois (the only state boards in existence at that date). The *Report* for 1884 of the Illinois Board of Public Charities (chap. iii, p. 65) has a very full summary of the subject from the pen of Secretary Wines (see paper, "Development of State Hospital at Kankakee," *Journal of the American Medical Association*, June 10, 1916).

come in any event but was helped decisively by this experiment. Diversified quarters adapted to the care of different classes of patients came to be required as a matter of course.

A subject of great interest in the management of mental patients was that of mechanical restraint, then in general use, by means of various forms of apparatus—straight waistcoats, leather muffs, anklets, bed straps. These had been considered necessary in the early days almost as a matter of course, in cases of maniacal or violent patients. Occasional emergencies, indeed, rendered them positively necessary; and the idea of demoniacal possession still influenced the minds of attendants, to whom milder methods would have seemed absurd. There is proof, indeed, that restraint was advocated by medical men as a mode of treatment at that time; that it was regarded as salutary by high authority, even by Dr. Isaac Ray, and by Dr. John P. Gray, of Utica Asylum, who permitted the use of the "crib bedstead" with cover that could be fastened down. A contest was waged for non-restraint and disuse of mechanical devices, from about 1870 to the beginning of the twentieth century, when general agreement was reached as to abolition of them except in emergencies, for it was seen that the method itself was at fault, often causing the trouble it sought to deal with. An era of greater freedom, quiet, and comfort descended. In abolishing restraint at Kankakee, I had all apparatus removed from the wards and stored in the dispensary. If an attendant or nurse thought restraint or seclusion necessary, he or she was obliged to report the fact to the doctor in charge. The doctor investigated; and if satisfied such measure was necessary, he had the restraint or seclusion applied in his presence, gave direction as to the length of time it should be used, and required that the apparatus be returned or the seclusion ended at the time specified. A record was kept of each case in which restraint was used.

The formal training of the attendants and nurses employed in the care of mental patients was a process of slow and difficult development. It was, in the first place, not easy to secure persons having the desirable qualifications who would be willing to become caretakers of individuals deprived of reason. A strong prejudice, based upon unfamiliarity and exaggerated fears, would need to be overcome. The compensation offered was not such as to attract very capable persons. This was true in a lesser degree in that day, of even those who would engage for service in the care of ordinary sickness in the general hospitals. It is not strange, then, that almost the only desirable persons who would at first take such service did so from religious motives. It was mainly the daughters of the church, Catholic and Protestant Sisters of Charity, who possessed both the desirable qualities and the willingness for such service. The men and women who applied for work as attendants in the institutions for insane in the 1870's often were illiterate, ignorant, even harsh and abusive.

Development of training schools for mental nursing followed in the wake of training schools in the general hospitals; and although later in realization, it is worthy of note that the impetus for training nurses in England and America originated with Florence Nightingale. She in turn derived her inspiration from visiting the Institute of Protestant Deaconesses at Kaisersworth, established by Pastor Fliedner. There she took a regular course of training; gained experience with all forms of sickness, including psychoses, in an asylum for female mental patients. The Deaconesses were a religious order like the Catholic Sisters, but did not make their vows for life. The work of the sisterhoods, undertaken from high motives, was excellent; but the supply of such nurses could never equal the demand. The compensation afforded by the public institutions would not be such as to attract persons of skill or ability, who could demand better pay or more attractive positions. This low wage standard seemed to be an insurmountable barrier to obtaining the desired order of nurses; and it continued to be so until the idea of instruction and training within the institution finally took root. Beginning with a book of rules, Conolly published *Teachings for Attendants;* and within a few years every hospital had its rules and regulations, its talks and lectures; even quizzes were given. All of this was preliminary to the first actual school, created by Edward Cowles at the McLean Hospital in 1882,[19] which was complete in form, with principal, instructors, and an elementary course in psychoses, courses in general and surgical nursing being given in affiliation with the Massachusetts General Hospital. Other training schools soon came into being: In 1885 Granger organized a school at Buffalo; Fletcher, at Indianapolis; Dewey, at Kankakee; Wise, at Willard; Hinkley, at Essex established schools in 1888 and 1889. Dr. C. P. Bancroft at Concord, New Hampshire, and Dr. C. W. Page at Middletown, Connecticut followed; and in 1894, Dr. C. B. Burr had a training-school at Flint, Michigan. There are today over sixty such

[19] Article by Edward Cowles in Tuke's *Dictionary of Psychological Medicine* (Philadelphia: Blackiston & Son, 1892). Even earlier, Bell and Woodward, in this country, issued: *Directions for Attendants.* Similar books were later issued by Kirkbride, Curwen, and Ray. An excellent *Handbook for Instruction of Attendants,* prepared by a committee of the British Medico-Psychological Association, appeared in 1885. Also in the early eighties an excellent little manual by W. D. Granger, of the Buffalo State Hospital.

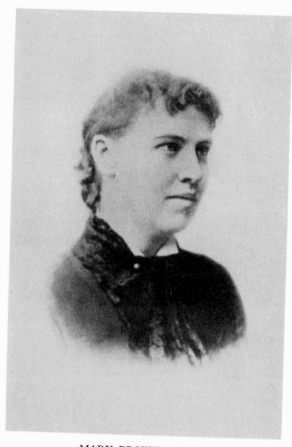

MARY BROWN DEWEY

schools that have been standardized under the rules of the American Psychiatric Association. At Kankakee a class of thirty-six was graduated in 1888, after a two-year course of training, and thereafter regularly until 1892, when a political turnover in Illinois brought about many changes.

In 1886 I was married to Mary E. Brown, of Brighton, New York, a graduate in nursing and in medicine, who had, with marked success, organized the first training school for nurses west of New York State, at the County Hospital, in Chicago. Her assistance in planning the course for nurses and attendants at Kankakee was invaluable. In this course an effort was made to influence the attitude of the attendants toward those in their charge. The lines from Matt. 25: 32-40 were quoted in the Book of Rules, and the following comment appended: "The above words, taken from the account of the Last Judgment, well express the work which falls to the lot of those employed in a Hospital for Mental Diseases; for within these walls are hungry to be fed, the naked to be clothed, strangers to be received and welcomed; those who are sick and imprisoned (by illness) are to be visited. This work has need of all the kindness, gentleness and unselfishness of which we are capable." Emphasis was placed upon the peculiar needs of those sick in mind, and upon the requirement that the patient, though removed from home, should have in the hospital whatever of homelike comfort and consideration was still possible.

In this connection should be named two of the great agencies for cure: occupational therapy and hydrotherapy. Pages would be required to tell of the use through the former of hours otherwise void—and, more important, to tell of the attainment of its great object, giving to aimless hands and minds the boon of creative effort; giving to lives joyless and unprofitable the glow of returning purpose and interest. Of hydrotherapy, the manifold application of water in the treatment of psychoses, it is scarcely necessary to write. The world knows of the beneficent effects of prolonged warm baths, sprays, the dripping sheet, packs hot and cold, which have removed the need of coercion; knows, too, of the healing use of electric current, violet ray, and massage.

In 1891, through the influence of one of the trustees of the institution, Mr. Ezra B. McCagg, of Chicago, a gift was made to the Hospital by the artist George P. Healy, of seventy-one of his paintings, portraits and landscapes. The collection was on exhibition for a time in our new "Amusement Hall" before being distributed among the wards and buildings of the institution. The following lines are a portion of a letter written by me to Mr. Healy in acknowledgment of

his gift: "Our only regret is that all our other pic-
tures are scarcely to be enjoyed any more. . . . .
We are proud to have your assistance in our work
of healing and beguiling disordered minds; it is an
honor to you that you preferred bestowing this
wealth on the needy and helpless to lift them up
by the power of your genius. . . . . You have conferred upon this Hospital a great distinction; to
my knowledge there are but two that possess
any important work of a painter of the first rank:
at Worcester, Massachusetts, in the chapel, there
is a painting of Allston's, also some good portraits of Miss Dorothea Dix; and there is at
Indianapolis a good copy of 'Pinel à la Salpêtrière'; that is all. Kankakee has therefore a great
distinction. . . . . This rich treasure will be care-
fully guarded, and will make your name familiar
and beloved here for all time to come."

John P. Altgeld, candidate of the Democratic
party, was elected governor of Illinois in 1892,
and on taking office, made a clean sweep of the
office-holders of the state in favor of those of his
own party. As a result, Dr. S. V. Clevenger, of
Chicago, a physician of good standing as neurologist and psychiatrist, was appointed as successor to myself as medical superintendent of the
State Hospital at Kankakee.

Governor Altgeld was an able lawyer of character, courage, and independence, somewhat giv-

en to demagoguery. The following lines from a poem by Edgar Lee Masters in his *Spoon River Anthology* describe the impression made by Altgeld during his campaign for the governorship:

> Tell me, was Altgeld elected Governor?
> For when I saw him
> And took his hand,
> The child-like blueness of his eyes
> Moved me to tears.
> And there was an air of eternity about him,
> Like the cold clear light that rests at dawn
> On the hills.

That the new governor possessed ample courage and self-reliance none could deny, whether approving or not of his acts and opinions. He did not hesitate to rebuke President Cleveland during the strike riots in 1894 for sending federal troops to see that the mails were not interrupted; the President, he declared, had trespassed upon his prerogatives as governor. Altgeld pardoned the so-called "anarchists," Fielden, Schwab, and Neebe, who had been seven years in the penitentiary after their co-conspirators, Parsons, Engel, Spies, and Fisher were hanged in 1887, following the Haymarket Riot. All his sympathy was with the "underdogs, unconstitutionally found guilty of conspiracy to murder a policeman," he maintained. He was, no doubt, desirous of good service in the institutions of the state;

but the appointments of trustees made by him, and the power placed in the hands of persons unfit to use it, resulted in confusion and scandal, as the sequel showed.

From a book entitled *The Don Quixote of Psychiatry*[20] by S. V. Clevenger (my successor) and Victor Robinson, I quote the following description of the Hospital at Kankakee:

The largest institution of the kind in Illinois,
The second largest in the United States.
Forty acres covered with buildings,
Eight hundred acres under cultivation.
Herds of cattle—
The nurses and training school students
Three hundred attendants; one thousand male patients,
One thousand female patients, ...

Dr. J. G. Kiernan, of Chicago, informed the writer that the position at Kankakee was first offered to himself, and he declined, saying, "To displace the present superintendent would be a blow to civil service." Dr. Clevenger states in the book above referred to: "Only when Dr. Dewey wrote that his relations with Kankakee were already severed, did I begin to consider the matter." Dr. Clevenger was a man of brilliant mind and ability as a physician, but the situation he encountered at Kankakee led in a short time to insurmountable difficulties. Immediately upon

[20] New York: Historico-Medical Press, 1919.

taking office he was instructed by a local political boss, now a trustee of the institution, and described by Clevenger as a "rascal," to appoint as business manager a man whom he, the trustee, had selected for the place, of whom Clevenger knew nothing. Soon he was required to appoint a storekeeper, selected in the same manner. Two of the three new trustees proposed the appointment of personal friends to fill important positions; the third, a saloon-keeper and brewer, sent his son with the following written request: "Anyting you can do for his founture wilfare will be appreviated by me" (*sic*). Dr. Clevenger's desire had been to observe civil service rules, but now he must either abandon his principles or antagonize his superiors. Checks made out ready for his signature, for thousands of dollars, in payment of bills of which he knew nothing, were laid before him by the bookkeeper. His refusal to sign led to "scenes" with the trustees; an atmosphere of distrust was created.

A serious source of disorder at this period was the invasion of the Hospital grounds on Sundays and holidays by crowds of excursionists. The Chicago papers advertised railroad excursions to Kankakee, giving the Hospital as an attraction. Sight-seers surrounded the buildings and gathered under the windows of the wards where the excitable patients were housed. Attempts to do away with these disgraceful scenes were not at first successful.

Dr. Clevenger became bewildered by these developments. He had near him no one upon whom he could rely; there appeared to be no good understanding anywhere; especially was he out of harmony with the trustees, who assumed control over appointments. His former experience with graft in the Cook County Asylum led him to suspect plots and wholesale plundering—even to the extent of believing that the railroad employees were removing carloads of coal from the Hospital sidetracks, in order to accuse him of complicity and theft. He proposed putting in lock switches and having the tracks patrolled at night.

Employees and officials of the former administration who remained had little sympathy with Dr. Clevenger; nor were those newly inducted in harmony with him; they were not of his choosing. His relations with the medical profession were impaired by his offering positions as consultants to ten of the leading specialists in Chicago, only to have the arrangement repudiated by the Board of Trustees. His attempt to exclude the excursionist visitors was regarded as autocratic. His many perplexities rendered him sleepless and nervous; having seen a superintendent of the Cook County Asylum assaulted, and having himself been fired at through a window, he grew apprehensive; his suspicions doubled. He remained in his house, with window blinds drawn.

The account in the book *Don Quixote* reads: "It was a wrecked Clevenger who walked the Hospital denouncing political graft." The trustees issued a statement in these words: "Owing to the overwork of Dr. Clevenger, it is considered advisable to give him a vacation of two weeks." The vacation was followed by permanent dismissal, and the comment in the book is: "It was an awful fizzle—ousted after three months, and nothing accomplished."

An event of importance during Dr. Clevenger's service was the appointment of Adolf Meyer as pathologist to the institution. Dr. Meyer had been referred to me by Dr. Ludwig Hektoen of Chicago before I resigned; and I, in leaving, earnestly recommended his appointment to Dr. Clevenger, who acted upon the recommendation. Dr. Meyer thus took the first step in his subsequent brilliant career. While at Kankakee he instituted many improvements in history-taking, joint consultations, clinics, and microscopic research. Also, he obtained valuable laboratory apparatus from the exhibit sent by the German government to the Chicago World's Fair in 1893.

The Association known now as the American

Psychiatric Association had its origin in 1844 under the name of the Association of Medical Superintendents of American Institutions for the Insane.[21] The first step toward united action was taken jointly by Dr. S. B. Woodward, of Massachusetts, and Dr. Francis T. Stribling, of Virginia. Being in agreement as to the need of an organization, they consulted one of their most influential leaders, Dr. Thomas S. Kirkbride, of Philadelphia; and a call was issued for a meeting to be held on October 16, 1844.

At this first meeting thirteen heads of institutions appeared. Six state institutions were represented: two of Virginia, Williamsburg and Staunton; one of Maine, Augusta; one of Massachusetts, Worcester; one of Ohio, Columbus; and one of New York, Utica. Four great charitable semi-public endowments were represented: Philadelphia's Pennsylvania Hospital, Providence's Butler Hospital, New York's Bloomingdale, Boston's McLean;[22] one municipal institution: the Lunatic Asylum of Boston; two private homes: Hud-

[21] The name of the Association was changed, at the fiftieth annual meeting in Washington in 1894, to the American Medico-Psychological Association; and again in 1921, at the seventy-seventh annual meeting, to American Psychiatric Association.

[22] Bloomingdale Hospital was and is the Department for Mental and Nervous Diseases of the New York Hospital. McLean Hospital was and is the Department for Mental and Nervous Diseases of the Massachusetts General Hospital.

son, New York, and Pepperell, Massachusetts. The thirteen members of this early Association I shall briefly characterize.

Dr. Thomas Story Kirkbride: Of the Pennsylvania Hospital, Philadelphia; pre-eminent constructor and organizer; author of the *Propositions*, the vade mecum of the Association for a generation; member of the Friends Society; friend of his patients in the truest sense, and devoted to their care for over forty years (1841–81); universally honored and beloved.

Dr. Luther Voss Bell: Held front rank in name and fame. "Bell's disease," first described by him was given his name. In medicine and administration he gained the highest distinction. In New Hampshire, his native state, his influence determined the creation of the State Hospital at Concord.

Dr. Pliny Earl: Accomplished in many branches of medicine; member of the faculty of New York College of Physicians and Surgeons; a great statistician; head of Bloomingdale Asylum for five years; leader of the onslaught which ended the immemorial custom of vicious bloodletting; able writer and reporter on developments in European hospitals; twenty years head of the State Asylum at Northampton, Massachusetts; like Dr. Kirkbride, a Quaker and a true friend of the insane.

Dr. Isaac Ray: National and international authority on medical jurisprudence of insanity; head of the State Hospital at Augusta; for twenty years in charge of the noble charitable endowment, Butler Hospital, Rhode Island; finally, for fourteen years an outstanding figure in medicolegal activity in Philadelphia; a writer of distinction. He bequeathed his estate to the work of Butler Hospital, and lies buried near by.

Dr. Samuel Bayard Woodward: His life was devoted to the care of the mentally ill. He and Dr. Eli Todd had a large part in the founding of the Hartford Retreat in 1824. Dr. Woodward was chosen as head of the first state institution of Massachusetts, and for fourteen years kept that hospital upon the highest plane. His influence determined the choice of his successor at Worcester, Dr. Chandler, and also gave to the city of Boston Dr. J. S. Butler, successful head of Boston's Lunatic Asylum.

Francis T. Stribling: Born in Virginia; a graduate in medicine of the University of Pennsylvania in 1830. He was superintendent of the State Hospital, at Staunton, Virginia, from 1840 to 1874. He exercised paternal oversight; encouraged occupation and diversion for patients; advocated parole or furlough. He and Dr. Samuel B. Woodward were the first to propose the Association of Superintendents; suggested it to Dr.

Thomas Kirkbride, who issued the call for the first meeting.

Dr. Amariah Brigham stands high in achievement for care of the insane. He administered the Hartford Retreat for two years, and in 1843 became head of the New York State Asylum at Utica. In his service at Utica he attained high excellence in medical administration and in deep study of the psychoses. Before the term "occupational therapy" was known, he practiced it with his patients out of doors and in. At Utica in 1844 he began the publication of the *American Journal of Insanity*, the second journal of its kind in the world. Dr. Brigham was an able and voluminous writer on the subject of mental disease.

Dr. John Minson Galt was another of the thirteen. He conducted the Williamsburg Virginia State Hospital with credit and success from 1841 to 1862. This institution, erected in 1773, was the first establishment for the insane on the American continent. Galt was a man of high character and scholarly attainments, being versed in European languages and in Arabic. His life ended tragically in 1862 with the occupation of Williamsburg by the Federal Army.

Dr. Samuel McClay Awl came as a pioneer from Pennsylvania to Ohio in 1826. He was at first interested in surgery; and in 1827, the first time "west of the mountains," he ligated the common carotid artery successfully in a child of eleven years; this operation had then been performed but three times in this country. He became a specialist in psychiatry; and when the Columbus State Hospital was opened in 1838, he was appointed medical superintendent. In 1835, with Dr. Daniel Drake, he founded the Ohio State Medical Society; through his influence a state institution for the blind was established in the late thirties.

Dr. John S. Butler, from his association with Dr. Woodward, acquired an interest in mental diseases, and was chosen in 1839 to superintend the Boston State Lunatic Asylum. Mr. Elliot mayor of the city, commended his "mingled kindness, care, and skill," praising him for vacating the previously existing "shocking cells" unfit for human habitation. His institution was visited by Charles Dickens, who in his *American Notes* expressed his warm approval on seeing the patients "sit down to dinner" with the doctor, and on seeing the doctor's wife, another lady, and two children "seated calmly among the women patients."

Dr. Charles H. Stedman, successor to Dr. Butler at the Boston institution, had entire charge of the hospital, the reformatory, the correctional and industrial institutions incorporated therewith, rendering valuable service from 1842 to 1851. He subsequently became one of the governor's council, and a member of the state senate in 1851.

Dr. Nehemiah Cutter, eminent in his profession at Pepperell, Massachusetts, received patients into his home, giving praiseworthy care for many years. He was interested also in educational matters, and largely supported Pepperell Academy.

Dr. Samuel White, from having a patient in his own family, came to give special study to mental disorders, and established a private institution in 1830. In 1840 he was elected president of the State Medical Society of New York, to which body he presented an address, summarizing the existing knowledge of mental disease, which was highly valued in his day.

The *American Journal of Insanity*, now the *American Journal of Psychiatry*, was established by Dr. Amariah Brigham at the State Lunatic Asylum at Utica in 1844;[23] and the first number appeared in July of that year. Dr. G. Alder Blumer well remarks: "It remains a monument

[23] The year 1844 saw three great national psychiatric journals come into existence: early in the year, *Allgemeine Zeitschrift für Psychiatrie;* in May, *Annales medico-psychologiques;* and in July the *American Journal of Insanity.* Within a comparatively short time (1848), two English periodicals devoted to psychiatry were published in London: the *Journal of Psychological Medicine* and *Mental Pathology;* Dr. Forbes Winslow was editor. In 1853 appeared the *Asylum Journal of Mental Science,* published by the English Association of Medical Officers of Asylums and Hospitals,

of Dr. Brigham's genius and energy."[24] The *Journal* was continuously published at the Utica State Asylum until 1894—after Dr. Brigham's death, in 1849, by his successors, Dr. Romeyn T. Beck, from 1849 to 1854; by Dr. John P. Gray, from 1854 to 1886; by Dr. G. Alder Blumer, from 1886 to 1894.

The members of the medical staff at Utica included many eminent psychiatrists: Dr. H. A. Buttolph, later head of two New Jersey state hospitals, in turn Trenton and Morris Plains; Dr. Van Deusen (who first described neurasthenia), renowned in Michigan as head of the Kalamazoo State Hospital; Dr. John B. Chapin, at the Willard New York Hospital, who built the first detached wards; Dr. A. O. Kellogg, renowned for his psychological studies of Shakespearian characters, who was consulted by Edwin Booth on Hamlet's mental state; Dr. Cleveland, head of the Poughkeepsie State Institution for twenty-six years; Dr. Judson B. Andrews, who, before serving on the staff of the Utica State Asylum, had done double service in the Civil War as captain of

and edited by Dr. J. C. Bucknill. Dr. Winslow's *Journal* was discontinued in its sixteenth year and was revived later under the name *Journal of Mental Science*. It is the property of the Royal Medico-Psychological Association. (From the Valedictory by Dr. E. N. Brush in *Journal of Insanity*, LXXXVII [N.S., Vol. X], 1061.)

[24] *Institutional Care of the Insane*, I, 75. Dr. Blumer, himself, continued in editorial charge from the death of Dr. John P. Gray in 1886 until 1894.

volunteers and as assistant surgeon, and who later was head of the Buffalo State Hospital (1880–94); Dr. Walter Kempster, who in 1883 was appointed superintendent of the State Hospital at Oshkosh, Wisconsin, and later was health officer in Milwaukee.

The years of Dr. Gray's editorship were marked by significant advance in brain pathology, microscopical study, and research. The members of the staff at Utica, all of whom as above mentioned, found distinguished service elsewhere, rendered important editorial assistance, and made significant contributions to the *Journal* in this period. In 1894 title to the *Journal* was acquired from the managers of the Utica Asylum by the American Medico-Psychological Association, and the *Journal* was transferred to Chicago for publication under the editorship of myself, who, with Edward Cowles and Dr. Henry M. Hurd, as a committee of the Association, were authorized to take this action. For three years I conducted the *Journal* in Chicago; but in 1897, owing to the double pressure of my Chicago practice and directorship of the Milwaukee Sanitarium, I submitted my resignation.

In 1897, the council of the Association formed an editorial board, consisting of Dr. Henry M. Hurd, as editor-in-chief, Dr. Alder G. Blumer,

Dr. J. Montgomery Mosher, Dr. Edward N. Brush, and Dr. C. K. Clarke, of Toronto. The Johns Hopkins Press assumed publication. For seven years, Dr. Hurd directed the *Journal*, with remarkable ability and success; it may be said of him: "Nihil tetegit quod non ornavit."

In 1898, at the meeting of the Association in St. Louis, there was presented to me in recognition of my services as editor, a *repoussé* silver pitcher. Dr. Richard Bucks, president of the Association, in making the presentation spoke as follows:

MY DEAR DR. DEWEY: I have the real pleasure and honor, on behalf of the Association, to present you with this pitcher, which we offer you as a very slight mark of the high esteem in which we hold you. We wish at the same time to express our deep sense of appreciation to the service you did us for three years as editor of the *Journal of Insanity*. This work you assumed and carried out ably and efficiently in spite of your other onerous employments. The Association feels that the work was performed by you at great sacrifice of energy which was otherwise needed by you, and in spite of that fact, was done in a manner which excited our deep admiration. In offering you this inadequate expression of our regard, we have also in mind your past services to our specialty as superintendent at Kankakee and as president of the Association in 1896.

In response I spoke in part as follows:

"MR. PRESIDENT AND FRIENDS: When I noticed upon the program the number that is now being carried out, I felt as if I might have to be carried out myself. The situation produced trepidation. I felt myself subject to abnormal manifestations. I could hear voices saying, "What have you done for the *Journal?*" and the answer, "Nothing to speak of." "What have you done for the Association?" and again, "Nothing, indeed." Bearing the name of an admiral[25] does not help matters in the least. It seems as if an explanation of the undeserved kindness and partiality shown to myself is to be found in the warmth and firmness of the bond that unites us as an Association. We occupy positions calculated in an especial manner to call out all the forbearance, loyalty, and good will of which we are capable. We are drawn to one another in keen sympathy and appreciation by the especial knowledge each one has of the toils and trials of the others, which only they can understand who are charged with the welfare of fellow-beings sick not only in body but in mind. Our duties are, not only medical and scientific, but humanitarian. I believe all the men who have won fame and honor in the care of the insane have been men of large and noble heart. I feel as if in this instance a part of your superabundant good will had been diverted toward myself; and although I may not deserve it, I accept it with deep thankfulness.

In 1904, when, after full measure of service, Dr. Hurd resigned from chief editorship of the *Journal*, his natural successor was Dr. Edward N. Brush, who could step fully equipped into this responsibility. Dr. Brush had had early experience as editor of the *Medical and Surgical Journal* of Buffalo from 1874 to 1878, had been on the

[25] Just at this time Admiral George Dewey had defeated the Spanish fleet and captured Manila.

staff at Utica six years, and had served seven years as assistant to Dr. Hurd at Baltimore. He held the chief editorship of the *Journal* with distinguished success for twenty-six years, until 1931. Dr. Hurd on resigning from the board of editors in 1911 was elected emeritus; in 1917, Dr. Blumer became editor emeritus. Dr. C. Macfie Campbell and Dr. Albert M. Barrett filled the vacancies.

Dr. J. Montgomery Mosher died in 1922. Aside from his fame as creator of "Pavilion F," he was clinical professor of psychiatry in Albany Medical College, and editor of the *Journal of Psychiatry*. "Pavilion F" was the department for mental and nervous diseases of the Albany City Hospital; it was the first psychiatric department to be built as a separate and independent unit for such diseases in connection with any American hospital,[26] and sprang entirely from the inspiration of Dr. Mosher. It has served as an incentive to the efforts of many others in this direction. Dr. George H. Kirby succeeded to the position of Dr. Mosher.

In 1921 the *American Journal of Insanity* became the *American Journal of Psychiatry*, and in 1927 it was decided the issues should appear bimonthly instead of quarterly. At this time, Dr. Harry Stack Sullivan and Dr. Clarence B. Farrar

[26] *American Journal of Psychiatry*, II, No. 4, 737.

became associate editors; and Dr. Karl Bowman, Dr. Henry A. Bucker, Jr., Dr. William Rush Dutton, Jr., Dr. Franklin G. Ebaugh, Dr. Theophile Ruphael, and Dr. Edward A. Stecker were made collaborators.

It was understood in 1931 that Dr. Brush contemplated retiring from the chief editorship of the *Journal*, and his colleagues desired to commemorate his retirement in a manner worthy of himself and his long service and to show their appreciation. Measures were taken for carrying out this plan. An illuminated scroll, inscribed as follows, was presented to him:

To Dr. EDWARD NATHANIEL BRUSH, Life member, and former President of the American Psychiatric Association, Distinguished physician, Administrator, Editor, Humanitarian—Homage from the Officers and members and from his colleagues on the Editorial Staff on the occasion of his retirement as Editor of the American Journal of Psychiatry, commemorating Forty years service on the Editorial Board, Twenty-six years as Editor-in-chief.

In appreciation of this unique service of untiring devotion and scholarship extending over so many years, and to express the high esteem and deep affection of his colleagues and friends, this scroll is presented at the eighty-seventh annual meeting of the American Psychiatric Association, held in Toronto, Canada, June first to fifth, 1931.

The scroll was signed by the president, vice-president, secretary-treasurer, associated editors, and collaborators.

A dinner was given on the evening of June 4; the president, Dr. English, presided.

In June, 1931, Dr. C. B. Farrar, the director of the Psychiatric Hospital of Toronto, was elected to the chief editorship of the *American Journal of Psychiatry*. Dr. Brush signified his enthusiastic approval of the selection. Dr. Farrar's attainments in psychiatry, his distinction and ability as a writer, and his highly successful career gave assurance of the continuation of the best traditions of the *Journal*.

TITLES OF PAPERS BY RICHARD
DEWEY, M.D.

1878 "Provision for Insane Criminals," *Chicago Journal of Nervous and Mental Diseases.*

1882 "Differentiation in Institutions for the Insane," *American Journal of Insanity.*

1884 "Congregate and Segregate Buildings for the Insane" (read before the Conference of Charities, 1884), *Alienist and Neurologist.*

1890 "Two Cases of Traumatic Injury of the Brain" (read at the annual meeting of the Association of Medical Superintendents), *American Journal of Insanity,* January, 1891.

"The Proper Disposition of the Criminal Insane," by Archibald Church, M.D., and Richard Dewey, M.D. (read before Chicago Medico-Legal Society).

1892 "Old and New Ideas with Regard to the Work and the Organization of Institutions for the Insane" (read before the Chicago Medical Society).

"Some Illustrations of the Working of the Plea of Insanity in Criminal Prosecutions: A Plea for Better Regulation of Expert Testimony" (read before Medico-Legal Society).

"Insanity Following the Keeley Treatment for Inebriety," *International Medical Magazine.*

1893   "The Proposed Legislation Regarding the Commitment of the Insane" (read before the Chicago Medico-Legal Society), *Journal of the American Medical Association*, April, 1893.

1894   "The Mental Condition of John Hart, the Double Sororicide," *North American Practitioner*.

1896   "Our Association and Our Associates" (address before Medico-Psychological Association, Boston, 1896).

1898   "Three Cases of General Paralysis in Husband and Wife," *Chicago Medical Recorder*, October, 1898.

"After-care of the Necessitous Insane," *American Journal of Insanity*.

1900   "Are There Any Conditions Which Would Warrant the Taking of Life Because of Incurable Mental Disease?" (read before the American Medico-Psychological Association, Richmond, May, 1900).

"Therapeutics of Travel and Change of Scene in Nervous and Mental Diseases" (presented to the Section on Nervous and Mental Diseases, Meeting of American Medical Association, June, 1900).

1901   "The Psychosis in Cerebral Syphilis" (read before American Medical Association), *Journal of the American Medical Association*, October, 1901.

"A Case of Masked Epilepsy with Criminal Complication," *Milwaukee Medical Journal*.

1903   "Therapeutic Notes," *American Journal of Insanity*.

"Apparent Recovery in a Case of Paranoia" (read before Medico-Psychological Association, May, 1903).

1904   "The Dividing Line between the Neuroses and the Psychoses" (read before the American Medical Association, June, 1904).

"A Case of Circular Insanity, Studied from Clinical, Differential, and Forensic Standpoints. With Gross and Microscopic Anatomy of Brain, from Pathological Laboratory of the University of Chicago, by Thor Rothstein, M.D., Chicago," *Journal of the American Medical Association*, April and May, 1904.

1905 "Clinical Report of a Case of Epilepsy; Malignant Tumor in Abdominal Wall; Hypodermic and Internal Nuclein Treatment; Subsidence of Tumor, and Incidental Remarkable Relief of Epilepsy for Seven Years since Treatment" (read before Chicago Medical Society, October, 1905).

1906 "Nervous and Mental Diseases in General Practice" (read before the Meeting of the State Medical Society of Wisconsin, June, 1906).

1907 "A Case of Disordered Personality," *Journal of Abnormal Psychology*.

1909 "A Case of Pseudo-coxalgia Relieved by Suggestive Therapeutics" (read before the State Medical Society of Wisconsin, at Madison, June, 1909).

1914 "Neuropathic and Psychopathic Hospitals with Reference to Medical Teaching" (read before the American Neurological Association, Albany, New York, May, 1914).

1915 "The Development of Detached Wards at the Kankakee State Hospital, 1880–1890" (read before the American Medico-Psychological Association, May, 1915).

"A Case Involving Differential Diagnosis between Paresis and Manic-Depressive Insanity (Expansive Form), in a Syphilitic Subject" (read before the Wisconsin State Medical Society, October, 1915).

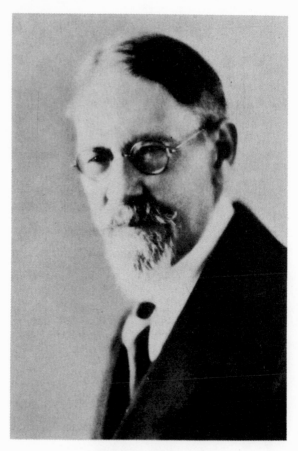

RICHARD DEWEY, 1932

1916   "Development of the State Hospital at Kankakee, 1880–1890," *Journal of the American Medical Association*, June 10, 1916.

1917   "Commitment to Psychopathic Hospital as Related to Question of Personal Liberty: Advantages of a Proposed Law for Detention Instead of the Existing Law for Commitment" (read before the American Neurological Association, May, 1917).

"Difficult Differentiation Diagnosis between Paranoia and Sanity" (read at meeting of alienists and neurologists, July, 1917).

1918   "The Nursing Problem as Related to Psychopathology" (read before American Medico-Psychological Association, June, 1918).

1926   "Assassinations and Sanity," *Pasadena Star-News*.

1927   "Early Days and Experiences in Psychiatry, 1870–1900" (read before Chicago Neurological Society, March, 1927).

1928   "Progress in State Care of Mental Diseases, Prior to 1900" (read at a joint meeting of the Society of Medical History of Chicago and the Institute of Medicine of Chicago, City Club of Chicago, March, 1928).

"Some of the Means for Guidance, Approach, and Appeal in the Psychoses" (read at the eighty-fourth annual meeting of the American Psychiatric Association, June, 1928).

"Comments on the Recent Census (1923) of the Insane in the United States" (not published).

"Mental Disease in the United States" (not published).

INDEX

⟦ PRINTED
IN U·S·A· ⟧

MENTAL ILLNESS AND SOCIAL POLICY
THE AMERICAN EXPERIENCE

AN ARNO PRESS COLLECTION

Barr, Martin W. Mental Defectives: Their History, Treatment and Training. 1904.

The Beginnings of American Psychiatric Thought and Practice: Five Accounts, 1811-1830. 1973

The Beginnings of Mental Hygiene in America: Three Selected Essays, 1833-1850. 1973

Briggs, L. Vernon, et al. History of the Psychopathic Hospital, Boston, Massachusetts. 1922

Briggs, L. Vernon. Occupation as a Substitute for Restraint in the Treatment of the Mentally Ill. 1923

Brigham, Amariah. An Inquiry Concerning the Diseases and Functions of the Brain, the Spinal Cord, and the Nerves. 1840

Brigham, Amariah. Observations on the Influence of Religion upon the Health and Physical Welfare of Mankind. 1835

Brill, A. A. Fundamental Conceptions of Psychoanalysis. 1921

Bucknill, John Charles. Notes on Asylums for the Insane in America. 1876

Conolly, John. The Treatment of the Insane Without Mechanical Restraints. 1856

Coriat, Isador H. What is Psychoanalysis? 1917

Deutsch, Albert. The Shame of the States. 1948

Dewey, Richard. Recollections of Richard Dewey: Pioneer in American Psychiatry. 1936

Earle, Pliny. Memoirs of Pliny Earle, M. D. with Extracts from his Diary and Letters (1830-1892) and Selections from his Professional Writings (1839-1891). 1898

Galt, John M. The Treatment of Insanity. 1846

Goddard, Henry Herbert. Feeble-mindedness: Its Causes and Consequences. 1926

Hammond, William A. A Treatise on Insanity in Its Medical Relations. 1883

Hazard, Thomas R. Report on the Poor and Insane in Rhode-Island. 1851

Hurd, Henry M., editor. The Institutional Care of the Insane in the United States and Canada. 1916/1917. Four volumes.

Kirkbride, Thomas S. On the Construction, Organization, and General Arrangements of Hospitals for the Insane. 1880

Meyer, Adolf. The Commonsense Psychiatry of Dr. Adolf Meyer: Fifty-two Selected Papers. 1948

Mitchell, S. Weir. Wear and Tear, or Hints for the Overworked. 1887

Morton, Thomas G. The History of the Pennsylvania Hospital, 1751-1895. 1895

Ordronaux, John. Jurisprudence in Medicine in Relation to the Law. 1869

The Origins of the State Mental Hospital in America: Six Documentary Studies, 1837-1856. 1973

Packard, Mrs. E. P. W. Modern Persecution, or Insane Asylums Unveiled, As Demonstrated by the Report of the Investigating Committee of the Legislature of Illinois. 1875. Two volumes in one

Prichard, James C. A Treatise on Insanity and Other Disorders Affecting the Mind. 1837

Prince, Morton. The Unconscious: The Fundamentals of Human Personality Normal and Abnormal. 1921

Putnam, James Jackson. Human Motives. 1915

Russell, William Logie. The New York Hospital: A History of the Psychiatric Service, 1771-1936. 1945

Sidis, Boris. The Psychology of Suggestion: A Research into the Subconscious Nature of Man and Society. 1899

Southard, Elmer E. Shell-Shock and Other Neuropsychiatric Problems Presented in Five Hundred and Eighty-Nine Case Histories from the War Literature, 1914-1918. 1919

Southard, E[lmer] E. and Mary C. Jarrett. The Kingdom of Evils. 1922

Southard, E[lmer] E. and H[arry] C. Solomon. Neurosyphilis: Modern Systematic Diagnosis and Treatment Presented in One Hundred and Thirty-seven Case Histories. 1917

Spitzka, E[dward] C. Insanity: Its Classification, Diagnosis and Treatment. 1887

Supreme Court Holding a Criminal Term, No. 14056. The United States vs. Charles J. Guiteau. 1881/1882. Two volumes

Trezevant, Daniel H. Letters to his Excellency Governor Manning on the Lunatic Asylum. 1854

Tuke, D[aniel] Hack. The Insane in the United States and Canada. 1885

Upham, Thomas C. Outlines of Imperfect and Disordered Mental Action. 1868

White, William A[lanson]. Twentieth Century Psychiatry: Its Contribution to Man's Knowledge of Himself. 1936

Willard, Sylvester D. Report on the Condition of the Insane Poor in the County Poor Houses of New York. 1865